Y0-AAX-999

ELECTRICAL STIMULATION OF THE HEART
IN THE STUDY AND TREATMENT
OF TACHYCARDIAS

ELECTRICAL STIMULATION
OF THE HEART
IN THE STUDY AND TREATMENT
OF TACHYCARDIAS

H. J. J. WELLENS M·D.

University Department of Cardiology (Director: Professor Dr. D. Durrer)
Wilhelmina Gasthuis, Amsterdam, The Netherlands

RC685
A65
W447e
1971

1971

UNIVERSITY PARK PRESS
BALTIMORE

265901

Copyright 1971 by H. E. Stenfert Kroese N.V., Publishers, P.O. Box 33, Leiden,
The Netherlands

Printed in The Netherlands by N.V. Drukkerij Batteljee & Terpstra, Leiden

Library of Congress Catalogue Card number 74-153469

ISBN 0.8391.0602.5

All rights reserved.

No part of this book may be reproduced by print, photoprint, or any other means
without written permission of the publisher.

To the memory of my father
To Inez

CONTENTS

INTRODUCTION

The interplay between the careful analysis of clinical electrocardiograms and results from animal experiments have in the past 60 years resulted in provocative and brillant concepts on the mechanisms of cardiac arrhythmias in man.

Many of the animal experiments however were done on open-chested dogs with cut cardiac nerves and under the influence of pharmaca. It is doubtful, therefore whether these results can be transferred without reservation to the human situation.

The introduction of electrical stimulation of the heart in clinical cardiology has opened new ways to study some aspects of cardiac arrhythmias directly in the unaesthesized patient.

This study reports observations on patients who were admitted to the University Department of Cardiology, Wilhelmina Gasthuis, Amsterdam, for the evaluation and treatment of tachycardias. Electrically induced premature beats were used in an effort to elucidate the origin and mechanism of these tachycardias. The first chapter is on classification and diagnosis of tachycardias with special emphasis on our current knowledge of the differential diagnosis between supraventricular tachycardias with aberrant conduction and ventricular tachycardias.

This is followed by theoretical considerations on tachycardias especially in relation to the methods used in this study. After an outline of these methods the results of our studies in patients with atrial flutter, A-V junctional tachycardias and tachycardias related to the pre-excitation syndrome are reported. A discussion on the value of electrical stimulation for the treatment of tachycardias is followed by a summary of our results.

Several members of the University Department of Cardiology, Wilhelmina Gasthuis, Amsterdam, took part in the work reported here. The help of Dr. R. M. Schuilenburg has been indispensable. The study was inspired and expertly guided by Prof. Dr. D. Durrer.

The investigations were supported by a grant from the Netherlands Organization for the Advancement of Pure Research (Z.W.O.), the Hague, the Netherlands, and the Stichting Bijstand Cardiologische Kliniek, Amsterdam, the Netherlands. A generous gift from 'De Nederlandse Hartstichting' and 'De drie Lichten' enabled the publication of this study.

Figures 24, 32, 35 and 36 are published by permission of the Royal Netherlands Academy of Sciences. Figures 42 and 43 were reproduced from the American Journal of Cardiology (35) by permission of the publisher, Reuben H. Donnelley Corp., figures 46, 47, 48, 49, 50, 51, 53, 55, 56, 57 and 58 were reproduced from *Circulation,* by permission of the American Heart Association Inc.

CHAPTER 1

CLASSIFICATION AND DIAGNOSIS

OF TACHYCARDIAS

Despite the temptation of the cardioverter standing just around the corner, allowing immediate treatment of many tachycardias, the correct identification of the site of origin of a tachycardia (atrial, A-V junctional or ventricular) remains important for obvious etiologic, therapeutic and prognostic reasons.

This problem should be approached in a systematic way and requires the knowledge of:

1. a classification of tachycardias according to rhythm and rate, the relation between atrial and ventricular rhythm and their response to carotid sinus massage (CSM)
2. the characteristic signs on physical examination that accompany a certain type of tachycardia.

In this way the origin of the majority of tachycardias can be diagnosed. No verdict is possible however in those patients who present with a regular tachycardia, with an electrocardiogram showing wide QRS complexes without definite P waves, and who do not respond to carotid sinus massage.

The identification of the origin of these tachycardias is, to quote Marriott and Rogers,: 'the knottiest important quandary in the diagnosis of dysrhythmias'. For this group one has recourse to additional diagnostic procedures:

a. intra-esophageal and intra-atrial leads to identify atrial activity and its relation with ventricular activity.
b. the use of electrical stimulation of the heart to locate the origin of the tachycardia.
c. the recording of potentials from the specific conduction system.

CLASSIFICATION OF TACHYCARDIAS

As far as site of origin, atrial and ventricular rate and rhythm, and the response to carotid sinus stimulation is concerned, tachycardias can be classified as follows:

1. *Sinus tachycardia:*
Frequency 100-180/minute. Rhythm regular. Further increase in rate on exercise. On CSM gradual slowing of sinus rate with gradual increase in rate on termination of CSM.

2. *Atrial tachycardia:*
a. not related to digitalis medication:
   atrial rate 130-280/minute. Atrial rhythm regular. No change in rate on exercise. Frequently 1:1 relation between atrial and ventricular rate. On CSM no influence or abrupt termination of tachycardia.
b. resulting from digitalis intoxication:
   Frequency 130-250/minute. Atrial rhythm frequently irregular. Usually no 1:1 relation between atrial and ventricular rate, due to partial A-V block. On CSM decrease in ventricular rate from increase in A-V block.

3. *Atrial flutter:*
Atrial frequency 220-360/minute. Atrial rhythm regular. Ventricular rate and rhythm depend upon the degree of A-V block. On CSM:
a. usually decrease in ventricular rate due to increase in A-V block.
b. occasionally no effect.
c. rarely transition into atrial fibrillation.
d. very rarely termination of flutter, with appearance of sinus rhythm or A-V junctional escape rhythm.

4. *Atrial fibrillation:*
Atrial frequency 400-650/minute. Atrial rythm completely irregular Ventricular rhythm completely irregular. Ventricular rate depends upon A-V transmission. On CSM:
a. no effect.
b. slowing of ventricular rate due to increase in A-V block.

5. *A-V junctional tachycardia:*
a. non-paroxysmal. Ventricular rate 70-140/minute. Regular ventricular rhythm. Increase in ventricular rate on exercise. Atrial activation either retrograde from A-V junction or independent (A-V dissociation). On CSM no response or gradual slowing of ventricular rate.
b. paroxysmal. Ventricular rate 130-240/minute. Regular ventricular rhythm. Usually 1:1 retrograde conduction towards the atria. On CSM no response or abrupt cessation of the tachycardia.

6. *Ventricular tachycardia:*
Ventricular rate 120-210/minute. Ventricular rhythm regular or slightly irregular. Atrial rhythm either independent (A-V dissociation) or related to ventricular rhythm (retrograde conduction). No response to CSM.

7. *Circus movement tachycardias related to pre-exitation syndrome:*
Ventricular rate 140-260/minute. Regular ventricular rhythm. 1:1 relation between atrial and ventricular rhythm. On CSM:
a. no effect.
b. abrupt termination of tachycardia.
c. slowing of the tachycardia.

As far as we know slowing of the ventricular rate during carotid sinus stimulation in a patient with the WPW syndrome and a circus movement tachycardia has never been reported before. Figure 1 shows the effect of CSM during a tachycardia in a patient with WPW type A. The slight slowing in ventricular rate is probably caused by a decrease in conduction velocity in the A-V junction during carotid sinus stimulation.

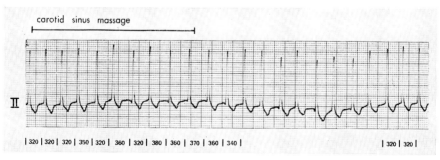

Fig. 1. Influence of carotid sinus massage on a tachycardia in a patient with Wolff-Parkinson-White syndrome type A.

Carotid sinus massage is of such diagnostic and therapeutic importance in patients with tachycardias, that it seems appropriate to include table 1 in this chapter. Even if properly done one occasionally has the startling experience that carotid sinus massage is followed by a long period of cardiac arrest, sometimes lasting more than 10 sec. Especially on terminating a tachycardia, and in patients older than 60 years of age, one should be prepared for such a surprise and have a fist ready to end the pause by a thump on the chest. At least three fatal cases of ventricular fibrillation following carotid sinus massage have been reported (Greenwood and Dupler (43), Porus and Marcus (115), and Alexander and Ping (2)). All these however were critically ill and received cardiac glycosides.

TABLE 1.   *Rules for carotid sinus massage (CSM).*

Precautions:
a. Try to exclude stenosis of one of the carotid arteries by palpation and auscultation.
b. Register the effect of CSM with help of an electrocardiogram; if not available, listen to the heart with the stethoscope during carotid sinus massage.
c. Realize that the older patient might respond with a long period of cardiac arrest.

Proper positioning:
a. Patient flat on his back with his head falling backward (either by placing the physician's left arm or a small pillow under the patient's shoulders).
b. Patient's head turned to the left during massage of the right carotid sinus, and vice versa.

Correct massaging:
a. On the bifurcation of the carotid artery just below the angle of the jaw.
b. Massage one side at a time.
c. Start by slight pressure (some, especially elderly, patients are very sensitive). Thereafter firm pressure should be applied with a massaging action.
d. Do not exceed 5 seconds at a time.

SIGNS ON PHYSICAL EXAMINATION

On physical examination of the patient with a tachycardia particular attention should be given to:
1. the first heart sound.
2. the jugular venous pulse.
3. the arterial blood pressure.

1. *The first heart sound*

It is obvious that an irregular tachycardia, with changing RR intervals (atrial tachycardia with block, atrial flutter with block, and atrial fibrillation) results in changing loudness of the first heart sound (although this may be minimal in patients with mitral stenosis).

Particular attention should be given to the first heart sound in patients with regular tachycardias. Marked and irregular changes in loudness indicate that no constant relation between atrial and ventricular contraction exists. This is the case when an independent ventricular and atrial rhythm are present during a ventricular or A-V junctional tachycardia. The atrial rhythm usually results from the sinus node but may originate in any ectopic atrial focus. A slow atrial rhythm facilitates the recognition of the changing loudness of the first heart sound. It is clear that no such changes are found when atrial fibrillation occurs during a ventricular or A-V junctional tachycardia.

In patients with dissociation between atrial and ventricular activity it is frequently possible to hear atrial sounds independent of the first heart sound. This strengthens the impression on auscultation that one is dealing with an A-V junctional or ventricular tachycardia with independent atrial activity.

2. *Jugular venous pulse*

Dissociation in atrial and ventricular activity results in changes in height and relation between A and V waves in the venous pressure pulse. When atrial contraction coincides with ventricular systole a cannon wave occurs. This knowledge can be used to diagnose independent contraction of atria and ventricles in patients with regular tachycardias. Again the two types of tachycardia creating this situation are the A-V junctional and ventricular tachycardia with independent atrial and ventricular rhythm. Of course these changes in venous pressure pulse are no longer present when atrial fibrillation occurs.

There is another situation where careful examination of the jugular venous pulse in patients with a regular tachycardia is of value. In patients with atrial flutter and 2:1 A-V conduction it is frequently possible to discern the flutter waves on inspection of the jugular vein.

3. *The arterial blood pressure*

Independent contraction of atrium and ventricle results in changes in atrial contribution to ventricular filling. Irregular blood pressure changes in patients with regular tachycardia, therefore, point to the presence of A-V junctional or ventricular tachycardia with independent atrial rhythm. This sign (151), easily recorded with the conventional blood pressure recording apparatus, is especially helpful in the sick patient with lowered blood pressure: It should be distinguished from alternating or paradoxic pressure changes. If atrial fibrillation occurs, this sign obviously disappears.

DIFFERENTIATION BETWEEN VENTRICULAR TACHYCARDIA AND SUPRAVENTRICULAR TACHYCARDIA WITH ABERRANT CONDUCTION

An important and frequently encountered problem in clinical cardiology is the patient with a regular tachycardia with a QRS complex measuring 0.12 seconds or more, without definite P waves. In this situation one has to decide whether this represents a true ventricular tachycardia or a supraventricular tachycardia with bundle branch block or aberrant conduction due to the functional properties of the bundle.

In the latter situation the impulse always arrives at the bundle branch (mostly the right one), when this is still refractory, resulting in persistence of aberrant conduction.

As stated before, a correct diagnosis is necessary for etiologic, therapeutic and prognostic reasons. From physical examination and a 12 lead electrocardiogram combined with carotid sinus massage, it is almost always possible to identify the patient with aberrant conduction during sinus tachycardia or atrial flutter.

Atrial and A-V junctional tachycardias can frequently be converted to sinus rhythm by carotid sinus massage.

The difficulty lies:

1. in the group of supraventricular tachycardias with aberrant conduction and independent atrial rhythm, versus the group of ventricular tachy- 1:1 retrograde conduction towards the atria.
2. in the group of A-V junctional tachycardias with aberrant conduction and independent atrial rhythm, versus the group of ventricular tachycardias with independent atrial rhythm.

Based upon the configuration of the QRS complex during the tachycardia, certain deductions as to the likelihood of a supraventricular or ventricular origin of the tachycardia can be made.

- In patients with a right bundle branch block pattern during their tachycardia a close look at lead V_1 may be rewarding. According to Sandler and Marriott (122) a mono- or biphasic pattern of the QRS complex in lead V_1 speaks in favour of a ventricular origin. A triphasic pattern would suggest a supraventricular origin with right bundle branch block.
- If one is lucky and has an ECG from prior to the tachycardia showing sinus rhythm, one has to look at the 0.02 sec. vector of the QRS complex in lead V_1. An identical initial vector, again according to Sandler and Marriot (122), would make a supraventricular origin of the tachycardia most likely.
- When during sinus rhythm ventricular premature beats were present, a configuration of the QRS complex during the tachycardia identical to these ventricular premature beats, argues for a ventricular origin of the tachycardia.

Dissociated activity of atrium and ventricle has for a long time been considered the hall-mark of ventricular tachycardia. It was realized that this dissociation is usually caused, not by antegrade A-V block, but by the rapid ventricular rate reducing the change for a supraventricular impulse after traversing the A-V junction, to find the ventricular myocardium responsive to stimulation. The occasional occurrence of such an antegrade conducted impulse leads to a 'capture' beat or a fusion complex between such a 'capture' and ectopic ventricular beat. Much emphasis has been placed on this finding in the diagnosis of ventricular tachycardia. One should realize, however:

- that smaller QRS complexes during a ventricular tachycardia do not only result from antegradely conducted 'capture' beats or fusion with 'capture' beats, but also from fusion with ventricular premature beats arising in the contralateral ventricle and reciprocal ventricular beats (Malinow and Langendorf (86), Latour et al. (71), and Vermeulen and Wellens (141).
- Fusion beats have also been demonstrated to occur between two supraventricular impulses with one of them travelling aberrantly by way of a preferential pathway (Kistin 1966 (64)).

The introduction of esophageal (Brown 1936 (9)) and intra-atrial leads (Hecht 1946 (50)) has markedly facilitated the study of the relations between atrial and ventricular activity during tachycardias. Kistin and coworkers (Kistin 1961 (63) and Kistin et al. 1967 (65)) have shown that retrograde

A-V conduction during ventricular tachycardia is quite common, frequently in a 1:1 way.

It was also demonstrated that atrial activation is in a caudo-cranial direction. This brings us to the problem that when a wide QRS complex, a 1:1 relation between atrial and ventricular activity, and atrial activation in a caudo-cranial direction, are present during a tachycardia, four possibilities as to the origin of the tachycardia exist:

1. atrial tachycardia with aberrant conduction. The atrial focus must then be situated low in the atrium;
2. A-V junctional tachycardia with aberrant conduction and retograde A-V conduction;
3. circus movement tachycardia (related to the pre-excitation syndrome) with aberrant conduction (either due to antegrade His conduction with bundle branch block, or antegrade conduction through the anomalous pathway);
4. Ventricular tachycardia with retrograde A-V conduction.

The introduction of electrical stimulation of the heart and the recording of potentials from the specific conduction system have opened new ways to solve this often perplexing riddle.

HIS BUNDLE RECORDINGS

In 1958 Alanis et al. (1) recorded the electrical activity of the His bundle in the dog heart. Giraud, Puech and Latour (41) were the first to record these potentials in man during catheterization of the right side of the heart. Scherlag and coworkers (129) have introduced a method to record His' bundle activity in man in a systematic reproducible way. They showed that normally His bundle activity is located 30 to 55 msec before the QRS complex. Using this approach A-V conduction and heart block in man was studied (Damato et al. 1969 (26)). The same authors also showed the value of His bundle recordings in the differentiation between aberrant conduction and ventricular premature beats in patients with atrial fibrillation (Lau et al. (72)).

If during a tachycardia one uses the presence or absence of a His bundle complex preceding the QRS complex as the dividing line between a supraventricular or ventricular origin, one has to redefine ventricular tachycardia.

The term 'ventricular tachycardia' should then be restricted to those tachycardias originating in the ventricle outside or below the His bundle.

ELECTRICAL STIMULATION OF THE HEART

As will be shown in succeeding chapters, the registration of the influence of electrically induced premature beats on the tachycardia allows conclusions to be made about the site of the ectopic focus.

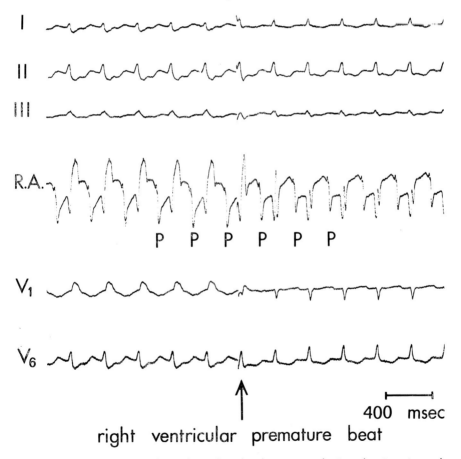

Fig. 2. Supraventricular tachycardia with right aberrant conduction due to retrograde invasion into the right bundle branch. The sequence of retrograde invasion into the right bundle branch causing functional right bundle branch block is interrupted by one electrically induced right ventricular premature beat, see Wellens and Durrer (144).

A ventricular tachycardia cannot be terminated by one or two atrial premature beats. Neither can an atrial tachycardia be ended with one or two ventricular premature beats (see fig. 26). The influence of atrial and ventricular premature beats on A-V junctional tachycardias is a complex one, as will be shown in chapter 5.

Sometimes during a tachycardia the wide QRS complex is caused by retrograde invasion into one of the bundle branches causing functional bundle branch block (Moe et al. (101), Wellens and Durrer, (144)). This sequence of retrograde invasion maintaining a wide QRS complex can be interrupted by one fortuitously timed ventricular premature beat. This immediately results in the emergence of small QRS complexes during the tachycardia, revealing its supraventricular origin (Wellens and Durrer (144)). (See also fig. 2)

DIFFERENTIATION BETWEEN A-V JUNCTIONAL TACHYCARDIA WITH ABERRANT CONDUCTION AND INDEPENDENT ATRIAL ACTIVITY, AND VENTRICULAR TACHY-CARDIA WITH INDEPENDENT ATRIAL ACTIVITY

Again recording the His bundle potential and the use of electrically induced premature beats, are of value in differentiating between an A-V junctional and a ventricular origin.

Another method to distinguish between these two was suggested by Easly and Goldstein (36). They assumed that, if in patients with aberrant conduction, atrial pacing would result in 'captured' beats, these beats would have a configuration identical to the tachycardia complexes. Theoretically this assumption is not a correct one. Depending upon the functional characteristics of the A-V junction and upon the prematurity of the electrically induced atrial beat, this beat, if it passes the A-V junction, will arrive at the junction of the bundle branches (1) earlier (2), at about the same time, or (3) later than the expected time of arrival of the impulse of the tachycardia.

In situation (1) the induced atrial beat might also find the other bundle branch refractory, resulting in bilateral bundle branch block and no QRS complex will follow the induced P wave. In siutation (2) the induced atrial beat will be followed by the same degree of aberrant conduction as shown by the tachycardia complexes. In situation (3) one has to assume that after discharging the ectopic supraventricular focus a marked delay in conduction of the prematurely induced atrial impulse takes place in the A-V junction, resulting in late arrival at the junction of the bundle branches. If both bundle branches have recovered at that time, such a 'delayed capture', (a term introduced by Pick and Dominguez (111) would be followed by a QRS complex of normal width. The occurrence of less aberrant or non-aberrant conduction following atrial pacing can therefore not be used as a conclusive argument for a ventricular origin of the tachycardia.

What will happen during atrial pacing in a patient where the aberrant conduction during a supraventricular tachycardia is caused by a functional bundle branch block by retrograde invasion into one of the bundle branches? (Wellens and Durrer (144)).

Under these circumstances an atrial 'capture' could disrupt the delicate time relations necessary for maintaining the functional bundle branch block. Such an atrial 'capture' would then be followed by a change in QRS complex configuration during the tachycardia from wide to small ones.

SUMMARY

In this chapter we gave a classification of the tachycardias. Signs on physical examination that can be of help in the diagnosis of tachycardias were reviewed.

The difficult problem in the diagnosis of clinical tachycardias is the differentiation between supraventricular tachycardias with wide QRS complexes and ventricular tachycardias.

The introduction of His bundle recordings and the response to electrical stimulation of the heart have opened new ways for the identification of the site of origin of these tachycardias.

CHAPTER 2

TACHYCARDIAS

THEORETICAL CONSIDERATIONS

Hoffman (53), Watanabe and Dreifus (143), and Singer and Ten Eyck (134) have recently reviewed our present concepts on cardiac arrhythmias. But, to quote Hoffman,: 'The information derived from experiments, which forms the basis of our ideas concerning the genesis of cardiac arrhythmias is known to be valid only for isolated preparations of cardiac tissue or in some instances for the normal in situ canine heart'.

This means that our knowledge on clinical arrhythmias is based on indirect evidence and therefore largely speculative.

This study is restricted to selected regular tachycardias in the human heart (atrial flutter, A-V junctional tachycardia and tachycardias related to the pre-excitation syndrome).

Regular tachycardias have been considered as either

1. arising in a rapidly discharging focus or
2. resulting from a re-entry or reciprocal mechanism, leading to a circus movement tachycardia.

Focal tachycardias have been divided into those caused by an unprotected focus and those resulting from a protected one.

In our patients electrically induced atrial and ventricular premature beats were used to initiate and terminate tachycardias, and to study the influence of a premature beat on the time relations of the tachycardia. The aims were:

1. The clarification of some of the mechanisms (focal vs reciprocal) of a tachycardia.
2. The localization of the site of origin of the tachycardia.
3. The evaluation of the value of induction of premature beats for the treatment of tachycardias.

INITIATION OF TACHYCARDIAS

We know that many factors promote and influence enhanced normal and abnormal focal impulse formation in the heart (see the articles referred to at the beginning of this chapter).

But although it has been demonstrated to occur in the digitalized human heart (Lown et al. (84) and believed to happen in the 'normal' heart (Scherf et al. (126)) we do not know the exact mechanism by which rapid automaticity develops after a single premature beat. The initiation of tachycardia by a single premature beat is much easier to understand if one holds a reciprocal or re-entry mechanism responsible.

Contrary to a focal tachycardia which is caused by a disturbance in impulse formation, this type of tachycardia results from a disturbance in impulse conduction.

In order to initiate a tachycardia by a single premature impulse, one has to assume that this impulse in its course (through a proximal common pathway (PCP)) meets two divergent pathways with different properties (α and β) converging upon a distal common pathway (DCP). The premature impulse is blocked in one pathway (β), passes slowly through the other pathway (α), and is able to re-enter from the distal common pathway, pathway β at its distal end. By re-entering the now recovered pathway β, the

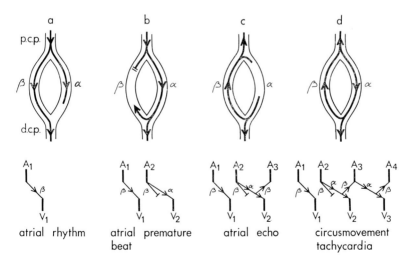

Fig. 3. See text for discussion.

impulse can be conducted back towards the proximal common pathway, giving rise to an echo beat, and to the proximal end of pathway α. Subsequent conduction through pathway α completes the first cycle of the tachycardia. Figures 3 and 4 illustrate how during atrial (A_1) and ventricular (V_1) driving a critically timed atrial (A_2) or ventricular (V_2) premature beat can initiate a reciprocal or circusmovement tachycardia. Essential is the presence of two pathways with undirectional block in one of them permitting re-entry in that particular pathway at its distal end (see also chapter 5).

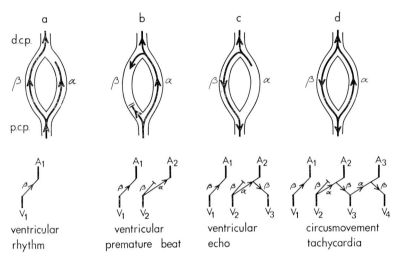

Fig. 4. See text for discussion.

This concept advanced as early as 1913 by Mines (96), can be used for the explanation of reciprocal tachycardias in the A-V junction (Scherf and Shookhoff (124), Moe and Mendez (103), Watanabe and Dreifus (143), and Durrer et al. (33)) and tachycardias in the Wolff-Parkinson-White syndrome (Wolff and White (153), Pick and Katz (118), Durrer et al. (31)). The concept can also be used for the explanation of atrial and ventricular tachycardias. Hoffman (53) demonstrated the possibility of re-entry at the junction between Purkinje fibers and the ventricular myocardium creating a pathway for a sustained ventricular tachycardia.

In all these types of tachycardias, the re-entrant activity leads to the formation of a circus movement (closed loop). As postulated by Moe et al. (101), another type of re-entrant activity generating ectopic impulses may occur. They observed in the dog heart that temporal dispersion in recovery of excitability takes place in ventricular muscle (Han and Moe (45). This finding could not be confirmed in the normal dog heart by Janse et al. (58).

There can be no doubt however that asynchrony of recovery of excitability in ventricular muscle increases on slowing of the heart rate, after ventricular premature beats and during myocardial ischemia. Under these circomstances re-excitation of already repolarised muscle fibers by fibers that are still depolarised might occur, leading to rapid repetitive ventricular responses.

It is obvious that the spatial dimension of the re-entry pathway present during a circus movement or closed loop tachycardia can differ considerably. Compare for instance the pathway for a reciprocal tachycardia in the Wolff-Parkinson-White syndrome with that of a ventricular tachycardia using two Purkinje fibers and a small piece of ventricular myocardium. This has important drawbacks on the influence of induced premature beats on a reciprocal tachycardia.

INFLUENCE OF INDUCED PREMATURE BEATS ON TACHYCARDIAS

Theoretically one would expect that the differences in causal mechanism of tachycardias can be studied by registering the events following an induced premature beat.

A tachycardia resulting from a protected ectopic focus which cannot be invaded and discharged by a premature stimulus would be characterized by a fully compensatory interval following the premature beat. Different results would be expected during a tachycardia caused by an unprotected focus or a re-entry mechanism. An early premature beat during the former would result in invasion and premature discharge of the unprotected focus.

Thereafter this focus would fire again at its previous rate, the post-premature beat interval being equal to or slightly longer than the tachycardia interval. In other words, during the tachycardia the post-premature beat interval would not fully compensate for the short interval, caused by the premature beat.

In the case of a re-entry or reciprocal mechanism one would expect that the premature beat will invade the re-entry pathway, resulting in shortening of one tachycardia cycle. The next cycle would then be equal to or slightly longer (since it is travelling closer to the refractory tail of the foregoing impulse) than the cycle length of the tachycardia. As mentioned before, the dimension of the pathway of tachycardias resulting from a re-entry or re-ciprocal mechanism, may differ considerably. If the dimensions are large, as has been postulated in atrial flutter, the same events will follow the in-duction of a single premature stimulus at two widely spaced points on the reciprocal pathway.

As far as the events following an induced premature stimulus during the tachycardia is concerned, it will be impossible however, to distinguish be-tween an unprotected focus and a small-sized re-entry pathway.

If these assumptions are correct, the systematic induction of premature stimuli to the heart during the tachycardia would enable us to unravel some of the mechanisms responsible for tachycardia. It should be stressed how-ever that in order to use this method correctly, the premature beat should be induced during the tachycardia after such an interval that the impulse can reach the focus or re-entry pathway before it will discharge.

This essential prerequisite is influenced by the following factors:

1. The frequency of the tachycardia and the resulting refractory period of atria and ventricles.
2. The distance between the site of the focus or re-entry pathway and the site of induction of the premature stimulus.
3. The conduction velocity of the exitatory wave in the area between the focus or re-entry pathway and the site of induction of the premature stimulus and vice versa.

Ad 1

An increase in frequency of the heart results in a decrease of the refractory period of atrial ventricular muscle. At frequencies above 100/min the re-fractory period in atrial and ventricular muscle measures roughly 40-50% of the cycle length, the percentage increasing with increasing frequencies.

The influence of fibrotic changes in atrial and ventricular muscle (for instance resulting from coronary artery disease or myocarditis) on the re-fractory period during the tachycardia is not known.

Changes in refractory period of A-V junctional tissue depend on the way the tachycardia is produced (Linhart et al. (80)). Exercise or adrenergic drugs result in shortening of the refractory period. Increasing the cardiac rate by electrical stimulation of atrium or ventricle leads to an increase in length of the A-V junctional refractory period. This knowledge is important for the understanding of the influence of electrically induced premature beats in A-V junctional tachycardias and reciprocal tachycardias using part or the whole of the A-V junction.

Ad 2 and 3

It is easy to understand that the longer the distance between the site of the ectopic focus or re-entry pathway, responsible for the tachycardia, and the site of electrical stimulation, the later it will be possible to elicit a premature beat. The time interval between the departure of the excitatory wave from the site of origin of the tachycardia till its arrival at the site of the stimulating electrode, will also depend upon the conduction velocity of the excitatory wave. These two factors also play a rôle in the arrival of the induced premature beat at the site of origin of the tachycardia.

The importance of these factors is demonstrated in figure 5. In this figure two stimulation sites (A and B) are shown at a distance of respectively *a* and *b* from the site of origin of the tachycardia. Let us compare the results of stimuli given at these sites during a tachycardia having a frequency of 150/min., and one with a frequency of 300/min.

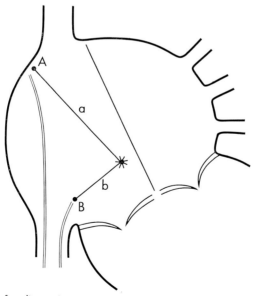

Fig. 5. See text for discussion.

Let us assume:
- That it takes respectively 60 and 20 msec. for the impulse to travel from the site of origin of the tachycardia to respectively point A and point B, and vice versa.
- That the refractory period during the tachycardia measures 50% of the tachycardia interval.

Tachycardia frequency 150/min.
(cycle length 400 msec., refractory period 200 msec.)

1. During the tachycardia the earliest possible premature beat can be given at site A 260 msec. after the origin of the tachycardia complex (refractory period + time necessary for the impulse to travel from the site of origin of the tachycardia to site A).

   This impulse will arrive at the site of origin of the tachycardia 260 + 60 = 320 msec after the origin of the tachycardia complex. This means that during a tachycardia with a frequency of 150/min., stimulation at site A will only enable one to study the influence of premature beats in the last 80 msec. (400 msec. − 320 msec.) of the tachycardia cycle.

2. The earliest possible premature beat can be given at site B. will be at 220 msec. after the origin of the tachycardia complex.

   This premature beat will arrive at the site of origin of the tachycardia 220 + 20 = 240 msec. after the beginning of the tachycardia complex. Therefore at this site of stimulation the interval during which we can study the influence of induced premature beats on the time relations of the tachycardia measures 400 − 240 = 160 msec.

Tachycardia frequency 300/min.
(cycle length 200 msec., refractory period 100 msec.)

1. The earliest possible premature beat that can be given at site A will be 100 + 60 = 160 msec. after the origin of the tachycardia complex.

   This stimulus will arrive at the site of origin of the tachycardia 160 + 60 = 220 msec. after the beginning of the tachycardia complex. At this time however, the next impulse of the tachycardia has already occurred (the tachycardia interval measures 200 msec.).

2. The earliest possible premature beat that can be given at site B will be 100 + 20 = 120 msec. after the beginning of the tachycardia complex.

This stimulus will arrive at the site of origin of the tachycardia $120 + 20 = 140$ msec. after the beginning of the tachycardia complex.

At this site of stimulation therefore the interval during which the influence of induced premature beats on the time relations of the tachycardia can be studied measures $200 - 140 = 60$ msec.

In these examples we assumed that velocity of impulse conduction between the site of origin of the tachycardia and the site of electrical stimulation stays the same during the two frequencies of the tachycardia. This is probably not true. Viersma (142) demonstrated in the isolated right atrium ol the rabbit that an increase in driving frequency results in a decrease in velocity of impulse conduction. Our own observations (Wellens and Freud (145) on the in situ right atrium of the dog heart are in agreement with this view. From our example (fig. 5) it is clear that at a frequency of 300/min. (as in atrial flutter) the premature stimulus given at site A will always on its way to the site of origin of the tachycardia, collide upon refractory tissue resulting from the next tachycardia impulse. Tachycardias originating low in the right atrium can be falsely considered to result from a protected ectopic focus when premature stimuli are induced only high in the right atrium. The same holds for right atrial stimulation during left atrial tachycardias. The importance of these factors becomes even more obvious during A-V junctional tachycardias where a focus or re-entry pathway is relatively protected by the properties of A-V junctional tissue.

It is understandable that in view of this complicating factors the use of premature stimuli will not always enable us to decide between a focal origin or a reciprocal mechanism in a certain tachycardia. We therefore also studied the way tachycardias could be initiated and terminated.

TERMINATION OF TACHYCARDIAS

Both Pick, Langendorf and Katz (109) and Dressler (29) gave clinical examples that cardiac pacemakers can be depressed by a single premature impulse. Lange (68) reported the effect of rapid ventricular stimulation on spontaneous pacemaker activity.

These observations suggest the possibility that a focal tachycardia can be terminated by one or two premature beats.

The actual mechanism at the cellular level responsible for this phenomenon is not known.

It is much easier to understand how a reciprocal tachycardia can be terminated by way of a single premature beat. An appropriately timed premature beat given during the tachycardia would make part of the reciprocal pathway refractory, preventing the passage of the next circulating impulse, resulting in termination of the tachycardia.

Although as outlined above, there are clinical observations pointing to the possibility that focal tachycardias can be initiated and terminated by a single premature beat, experimental evidence for this assumption is urgently needed. We will therefore favour a diagnosis of reciprocal tachycardia if a tachycardia can be initiated and terminated by a single premature beat. As an additional argument for this diagnosis will be considered a non-compensatory interval following an induced premature beat during the tachycardia. As pointed out before, it is not always possible to induce a premature beat early enough and closely enough to the tachycardia pathway, to consider this finding essential for making the diagnosis of reciprocal tachycardia.

CHAPTER 3

METHODS

All patients were studied in the post-absorptive state. Unless specifically mentioned no patient received any medication prior to the investigation.

Using the Seldinger-technique two or more electrode catheters were passed under local anesthesia through one or both femoral veins and positioned under fluoroscopic control at the desired intracavitary location, usually the right atrium or the right ventricle.

Occasionally it was possible to reach the left side of the heart through an open foramen ovale. In two patients with W.P.W. type A concomitant mitral valve disease necessitated additional hemodynamic studies of the left side of the heart. In these patients a transseptal catheterization was performed. After the hemodynamic studies were done a fine bipolar electrode catheter was passed through the teflon catheter and advanced to the left side of the heart.

A bipolar catheter was used for electrical stimulation. A uni-or multipolar one was used:

1. for recording the intracavitary atrial or ventricular complex,
2. to identify the atrial rhythm, and
3. if possible to determine the direction of atrial activation.

In a few patients a tripolar electrode catheter was positioned over the tricuspid valve to record His bundle potentials (as described by Scherlag et al. (129)).

Electrical stimulation was done with help of a safe and accurate stimulator (31), designed and built by Prof. Dr. L. H. van der Tweel, Prof. Dr. J. Strackee and Mr. Leo Schoo (Laboratory of Medical Physics of the University of Amsterdam).

With this stimulator three independent stimuli (one driving stimulus creating a regular basic rhythm and two testing stimuli eliciting premature beats) can be applied either separately or combined. The stimuli are electrical current impulses that can be varied in strength and duration. The strength of the square wave-pulses is adjustable from 25 micro-A to 30 milli-A with a duration of 1, 2, 3, 4, 8 or 16 msec. Because the internal resistance of the stimulator is very high, the resistance of the tissue and the contact resistance of the stimulating electrodes have only a neglegible influence upon the strength of the stimulus. Each testing pulse can be presented after a chosen interval (accurate to one millisecond) and can be applied after each beat, every second beat, etc. up to once after every 16 beats.

The interval after which the testing pulse is applied can either be started by the driving stimulus or by feeding the electrical activity of the heart itself (as derived from a standard lead ECG or an intracavitary electrocardiogram) into a synchronizer. A blocking circuit in the synchronizer limits the upper frequency of the test pulses. Special care has been taken to ensure safety of the stimulator by preventing electroshock hazards (Burchell and Sturm (12), Starmer et al. (139)). By use of a transformer the current pulses are separated from ground guarding against unwanted dangerous interference from the mains. Spurious pulses, due to disturbances in the mains or the ground including on and off switching of the apparatus, are prevented. All stimuli as well as the electrical activity of the heart are displayed on the screen of an oscilloscope.

During this study the duration of the stimuli was kept at 2 msec. Current strength was less than two times the diastolic threshold current. (Van Dam et al. (24), Van Dam (25)).

A schematic representation of the way synchronization and stimulation were done (in this instance during the study of atrial flutter) is given in figure 6.

The protocol of the investigation in each patient depended upon whether they were studied during a tachycardia or during sinus rhythm. If a tachycardia was present (as in our patients with atrial flutter and A-V junctional tachycardias) the program consisted of:

1. Identification of atrial rhythm, its relation with ventricular rhythm, and if possible the direction of atrial activation.
2. The influence of one, if possible two, induced atrial premature beats on the time relations of the tachycardia.
3. The influence of one, if possible two, induced ventricular premature beats on the time relations of the tachycardia.
4. The result of driving the atrium at rates above the tachycardia frequency.

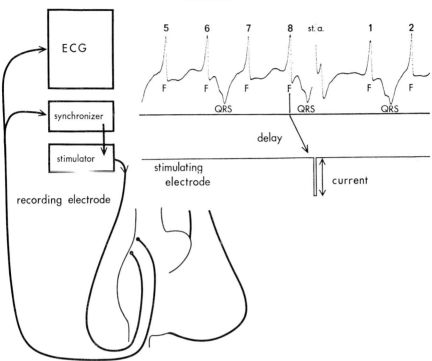

Fig. 6. Schematic representation of synchronization and stimulation as done in this study. This example is from a patient with atrial flutter. Two electrode catheters are lying close together in the right atrium. One catheter is connected both with the electrocardiograph, recording the intra-cavitary ECG, and the synchronizer. Using the top of the intra-atrial flutter complex for synchronization, an electrical stimulus can be given after the desired delay. Also the number of flutter complexes after one wants to deliver an electrical stimulus can be chosen. Shown here is a stimulus given after the eight flutter complex. The stimulus is delivered to the right atrium by way of the second electrode catheter.

If sinus rhythm was present (as in our patients with the pre-excitation syndrome), it was tried to initiate a tachycardia by:

1. Inducing one or sometimes two premature stimuli to the atrium after every eight beats of a regularly driven atrial rhythm. The premature beat interval was thereby gradually shortened, untill either a tachycardia resulted or the atrium became refractory to stimulation.
2. Inducing one or two premature stimuli to the ventricle after every eight beats of a regularly driven ventricular rhythm. Again the premature beat interval was thereby gradually shortened, untill either a tachycardia resulted or the ventricle became refractory to stimulation.

If a tachycardia resulted, the program outlined under tachycardia was followed.

Prior to the beginning of stimulation the position of the catheters was always controlled with help of the image intensifier. At the beginning of stimulation a drawing was made of the position of the catheters.

The results were observed in the ECG of leads I, II, III, V_1 and V_6 and multipolar intra-atrial leads.

In a few patients His bundle complexes were registered. The electrocardiograms were registered on an 8-channel high-frequency directwriting Elema recorder and stored on a magnetic tape with an Ampex FR 1300 tape recorder.

CHAPTER 4

ATRIAL FLUTTER

There is no unanimous opinion on the actual mechanism of atrial flutter in man. The two most favoured theories are: a circus movement, or a rapidly firing ectopic focus. Many experiments have been done in animal hearts to find evidence for either one of these hypotheses. (Lewis et al. (78), Rosen-blueth and Garcia Ramos (119), Scherf et al. (125), Brown et al. (8), Prinz-metal et al. (110), Lanari et al. (67) and Marques et al. (87)). These experiments however, can in many instances not be called realistic in the sense that their results can be transferred to the human situation. The presence of a safe and reliable electrical stimulator gave us the opportunity to study the mechanism causing atrial flutter directly in the human heart.

Our study was based on the assumption that atrial flutter would give a different post premature beat response, if the atrial flutter is caused by a circus movement or by a rapidly firing ectopic focus (see chapter 2).

Patients were only accepted for this study, if their conventional ECG's fulfilled the following criteria:

1. An atrial rate of at least 240/min.
2. F-waves, regularly spaced and equal in amplitude and contour.
3. F-waves, causing a continuous activity of the baseline.
4. On carotid sinus massage the characteristic sudden increase in flutter wave/ventricular complex ratio.

Clinical data on the six patients studied, are listed in table 2. Their ECG's are shown in figure 7.

Using the Seldinger technique two electrode catheters were passed through the femoral vein and positioned close together in the right atrium. One electrode catheter, a bipolar one, was placed against the atrial wall and used for electrical stimulation.

The other catheter, a multipolar one, was used for identification of the atrial rhythm. From one of the terminals of the latter electrode an intra-

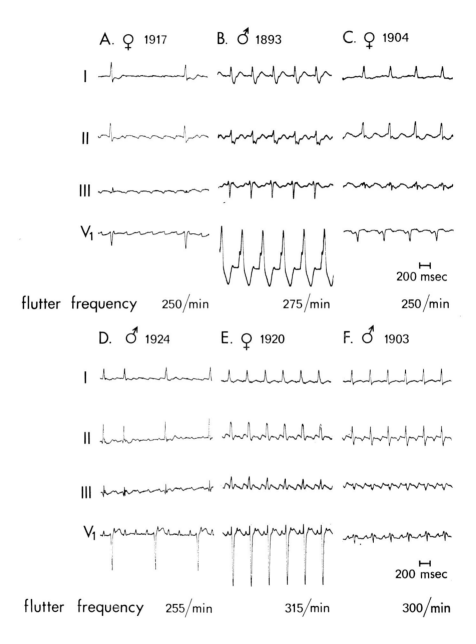

Fig. 7. Standard leads I, II and III, and lead V_1 of the six patients studied.

TABLE II

	Age	Sex	Diagnosis	Medication
Patient A	51	female	mitral stenosis aortic insufficiency	digitalis
Patient B	75	male	coronary artery disease	—
Patient C	63	female	mitral stenosis and insufficiency aortic insufficiency	—
Patient D	44	male	mitral stenosis and -insufficiency aortic stenosis and -insufficiency	digitalis
Patient E	48	female	pericarditis	—
Patient F	65	male	coronary artery disease	—

atrial complex was fed into the synchronizing circuit of our stimulator. Either one stimulus or two consecutive stimuli were given at chosen intervals once after every eighth flutter wave, using the top of the unipolar intra-atrial cavitary electrogram, derived from one of the terminals of a multipolar electrode catheter, for synchronization.

A schematic representation of the way synchronization and stimulation were done is given in figure 6. The protocol of the investigations was followed as outlined in chapter 2.

RESULTS

1. *Identification of the atrial rhythm*

On intra-atrial electrocardiography the 'flutter' complexes could be easily identified. In our patients the total width of the intra-atrial depolarization complex (as recorded from the right atrium) ranged from 75 to 150 msec. The smallest complexes were recorded in patients with the smallest atria. The intervals between 'flutter' complexes as measured from the intra-atrial recordings were not completely regular. Differences of 5-10 msec. were seen. This may be largely due to changing spatial relations between the atria and the catheter, under the influence of the movements of the heart.

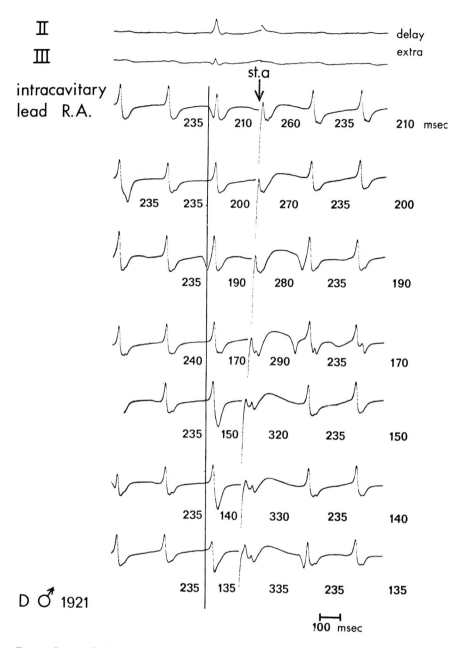

Fig. 8. Patient D. Intracavitary lead from the right atrium showing the pause following an electrically induced premature beat given high in the right atrium. On shortening the premature beat interval it becomes clear that the pause following the premature atrial activation is always fully compensatory.

2. *The influence of one electrically induced atrial premature beat on the atrial flutter*

Stimuli were applied high and low on the free lateral wall of the right atrium. The first site of stimulation was chosen to stimulate close to the origin of the reported internodal tracts (James (57) and Meredith and Titus (94)).

When an extra stimulus was applied to the atrial wall following every 8th flutter complex, and the interval between the last flutter complex and the extra stimulus progressively shortened up to the refractory period of the right atrium, the interval to the next flutter wave differed in length depending upon the site of atrial stimulation.

When the premature beat was given high in the right atrium, close to the superior caval vein, a fully compensatory or a slightly less than fully compensatory pause was seen following the extra stimulus. This was true up to the refractory period of the right atrium. Therefore the interval between the flutter wave preceding the extra stimulus and the following flutter wave

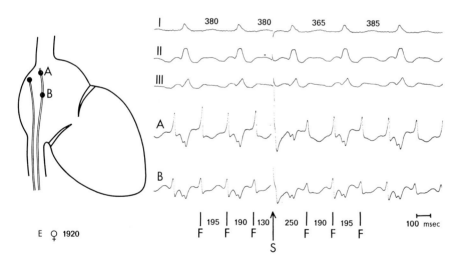

Fig. 9. Patient E. Influence of a premature stimulus given high on the lateral wall of the right atrium on the time relations of the atrial flutter. As shown in the intracavitary leads A and B the stimulus (S) is followed at the atrial level by a slightly less than compensatory pause. The standard leads show slight shortening of the interventricular interval (365 msec) following the R-R interval enclosing the premature atrial activation. This indicates that in this patient with 2 to 1 A-V conduction the first of the two flutter complexes is conducted to the ventricles. The drawing on the left shows the position of the stimulating and detecting electrode catheters. Only the right of the heart is shown.

was twice or almost twice the flutter interval. Figure 8 shows the fully compensatory pause following premature activation high in the right atrium during atrial flutter in patient D.

Figure 9 shows the slightly less than compensatory pause in patient E.

When however the premature stimulus was given low in the right atrium, a different pattern emerged. Now the extra stimulus was not followed by a compensatory pause, but by a flutter wave at a distance slightly longer than the flutter interval (fig. 10). In the presence of 2 to 1 A-V conduction during atrial flutter the changes in time relations of the atrial flutter following an atrial premature beat are nicely reflected at the ventricular level.

The RR interval following the RR interval enclosing a premature beat given low in the right atrium (fig. 10) is much shorter than when the premature beat is given high in the right atrium (fig. 9).

The sequence shown in figure 9 and 10 indicates that in patient E the first of the two flutter complexes was conducted to the ventricle. Is was never possible in our patients to stop the atrial flutter by a single electrically induced atrial premature beat.

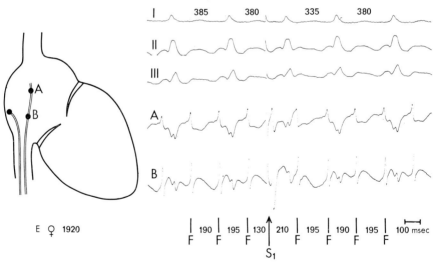

Fig. 10. Same patient as fig. 9. The influence of a premature stimulus given low on the lateral wall of the right atrium on the time relations of the atrial flutter. As shown in the intracavitary leads A and B a much shorter pause follows the premature stimulus as compared to fig. 9. The change in time relations of the atrial flutter is reflected at the ventricular level in shortening of the R-R interval following the R-R interval enclosing the premature atrial activation.

3. *The influence of two consecutive electrically induced atrial premature beats on the atrial flutter*

Similar to the findings listed under 2, the response to two successive premature atrial activations depended upon the site of stimulation. As shown in figure 11, two consecutive premature beats (S_1 and S_2), given high in the right atrium, were followed by a pause much longer than the flutter interval.

When however, the same was done lower in the right atrium the pause following the two premature beats was much shorter, being only slightly longer than the flutter interval (fig. 12).

It was never possible to stop the atrial flutter by two consecutively given atrial premature beats, not even at their shortest possible interval.

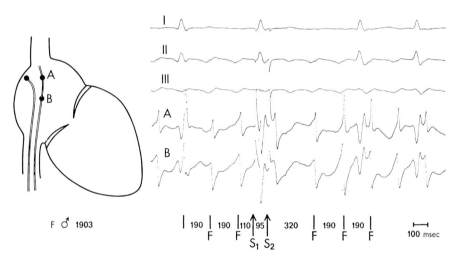

Fig. 11. Patient F. The effect of two successively induced atrial premature beats during atrial flutter. Points of stimulation high on the lateral wall of the right atrium. A pause much longer than the flutter interval follows the second premature activation.

4. *Results of driving the atrium at rates above the flutter frequency*

In three patients we drove the atrium at rates above the flutter frequency. This was done by regular driving of the right atrium with frequencies ranging from 300-400/min. This resulted in capture of the atrium by this higher frequency. When this rapid driving was discontinued the original atrial flutter readily emerged, the flutter interval being exactly the same as prior

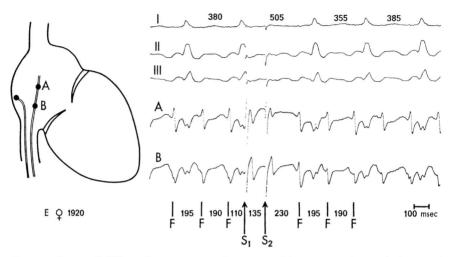

Fig. 12. Patient E. Effect of two sucessively given atrial premature beats during atrial flutter. Point of stimulation low on the lateral wall of the right atrium. The pause following the second premature activation is a little longer than the flutter interval. The R-R intervals show that this pattern of atrial stimulation causes 'concealed' A-V conduction.

to stimulation, the post stimulation interval being considerably longer than the flutter interval. An example is given in figure 13.

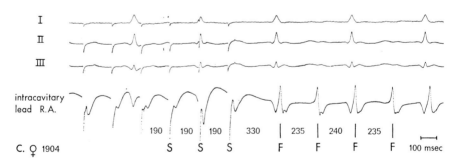

Fig. 13. Patient C. Effect of driving the atrium at rates above the flutter rate.
Point of stimulation : high on the lateral wall of the right atrium.
Driving Frequency   : 315/min.
Flutter frequency   : 250/min.
Driving results in capture of the right atrium. When driving is discontinued, the atrial flutter at its original frequency readily emerges. The post stimulatory pause is much longer than the flutter interval.

When the frequency of stimulation was further increased (more than 400/min) atrial fibrillation resulted. In two of our patients this was transient and followed after respectively 7 and 12 seconds by sinus rhythm. The latter has also been reported by Haft et al. (44), Lister et al. (81), and Zeft et al. (155).

DISCUSSION

In 1920 Lewis et al. (79) introduced the concept of a circus movement as the actual mechanism of atrial flutter in man. Since then other theories have been offered. From these the one that considers atrial flutter in man as caused by a rapidly firing ectopic focus has received most followers. Still both theories have enthusiastic advocates. This is well illustrated by two recent articles that review this subject extensively.

Rytand (121) closes his article with the sentence: 'The circus movement hypothesis appears to account for the mechanism of pure atrial flutter of the classical type'.

Scherf (128) summarizes: 'On the basis of the available data it must be concluded that experimental flutter can be caused by the rapid formation of impulses, whereas the theory of re-entry still requires proof. There is no definite proof for either mechanism in clinical flutter'.

Supporters of both theories have used intracavitary and intraesophageal leads to proof their point. An ectopic focus was favoured by Kossmann et al. (66), Coelho et al. (19), Prinzmetal et al. (116), and Latour and Puech (70). A circus movement by Steinberg et al. (140), and Rytand (121). Wenger and Hoffman (148), and Kishon and Smith (62) described two groups of patients, one where a circus movement was the most likely mechanism, and one where an ectopic focus seemed responsible for the atrial flutter. Katz and Pick (61) believe that both mechanisms may be correct for different types of atrial flutter.

In the distinction between the two mechanisms a long duration of atrial activity (as recorded intra-atrially), in relation to the total length of the interval between two flutter complexes, has been considered an argument for the presence of a circus movement during atrial flutter. One has to realize however that conduction velocity through the atrial wall is reduced at rapid atrial rates (Viersma (142)), and that pathology of the atrial wall is frequently present in patients with atrial flutter.

Intra-atrial leads, even multiple ones taken simultaneously with standard leads, have in our hands not been very helpful in solving the problem. Our difficulty was the exact location of the electrode catheter as far as its distance to the atrial septum and free atrial wall was concerned.

Very recently Rosen et al. (117) reported the close resemblance between atrial flutter and a unifocal tachycardia produced by rapid pacing from the coronary sinus.

They think that some cases of clinical atrial flutter may originate as a focal tachycardia from the coronary sinus or left atrium. Mirowski and Alkan (98), and Kishon and Smith (62) also believe that atrial flutter may arise in the left atrium.

A much more convincing method could be the mapping of atrial excitation during cardiac surgery in patients with atrial flutter. This has been done once by Hurley and Shumway (121). They concluded from their activation times that a circus movement was present in their patient.

We had the opportunity to study atrial activation in patient D when he was operated upon. Our results are in agreement with an ectopic focus, located low in the atrium. They will be reported in detail elsewhere (Wellens et al. (147)).

Our observations in patients with W.P.W. syndrome (Durrer et al. 1967 (31)) prompted us to tackle the problem from a different angle by studying the influence of induced atrial premature beats on the atrial flutter. As outlined in chapter 2, if one assumes that a circus movement, involving a large part of the atrium, is present during atrial flutter, stimulation of non-refractory parts of the right atrium, awaiting the arrival of the next flutter wave should either stop the flutter or shorten the duration of one cycle. The next interval should be of normal flutter cycle length. If conduction velocity and refractoriness are approximately the same in the upper and lower part of the lateral wall of the right atrium, premature stimuli given at these points after the same delay should lead to the same sequence of events. The detecting electrode should hereby lie close to the stimulating electrode (see fig. 14).

When an ectopic focus is responsible for the atrial flutter, this focus could either be protected (one that cannot be invaded and discharged by a premature stimulus (a parasystolic focus), or it could be unprotected, and be invaded and discharged by a premature stimulus (see chapter 2).

In the first situation premature atrial activation would always be followed by a fully compensatory pause. In the case of an unprotected ectopic focus,

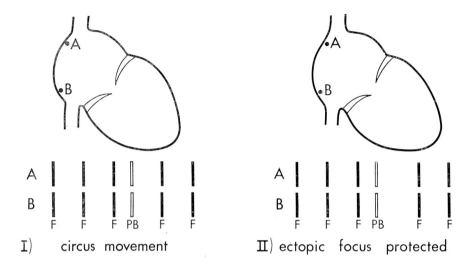

Fig. 14. Expected response to premature activation (PB) high (A) or low (B) in the right atrium in presence of a circus movement (I), a protected focus (II) or an un-protected focus (III) during atrial flutter (F-F).

I.   Premature activation of a part of the atrium participating in a circus movement should either stop the circus movement or shorten the duration of one cycle. The next interval should be of normal flutter cycle length. If recording and stimulating electrode are lying close together the sequence of events in this situation should be the same whether one stimulates at point A or point B.

II. If a protected ectopic focus were present the pause following the premature activation should always be fully compensatory, irrespective of the stimulation site. An interpolated beat is impossible due to the refractory period of the atrium.

a premature stimulus given close to the focus, would be able to invade and discharge the focus and to 'reset its time table'. The events following the premature beat would depend upon the time necessary for the premature impulse to travel over the right atrium to reach the ectopic focus (see also chapter 2).

If the unprotected focus were situated high in the right atrium, a premature stimulus given high in the right atrium would result in a much shorter post premature beat interval than when the stimulus is given low in the right atrium. The reverse is true for an ectopic focus located low in the right atrium (see fig. 14). In our patients who fulfilled Lewis' criteria (78) for the diagnosis of atrial flutter, premature activation of the right atrium during the arrhythmia never resulted in termination of the flutter.

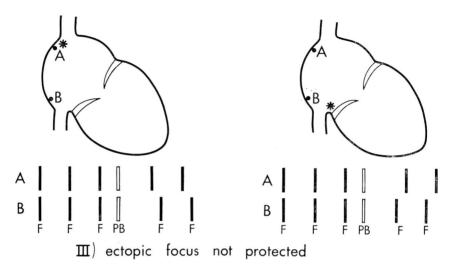

III) ectopic focus not protected

Fig. 14. continued
III. If an unprotected ectopic focus were present, the sequence of events is determined by the site of stimulation. If the stimulation site were close to the focus, the focus will be invaded and discharged early, resulting in a pause following the premature activation, slightly longer than the flutter interval. The pause following stimulation at sites further away from the focus. will depend upon the time necessary for this premature activation to reach the focus. An example of the effect of premature activation high (A) and low (B) in the right atrium in the presence of a focus situated high in the right atrium is shown on the left side of the figure.
The reversed situation is shown on the right side.

This was true both for one premature activation and two premature activations given in the closest possible succession.

Termination of atrial flutter and conversion to sinus rhythm by an appropriately timed electrical impulse delivered to the right atrium, was reported by Hunt et al. (55). This was observed when during the atrial flutter regular driving of the right atrium at a frequency of 180/min. was performed. From the figure accompanying the article it is very difficult to see what actually happened. In a later article from the same group (now headed by Zeft (155)) they reported on their experience in six more patients with atrial flutter where they drove the right atrium at 180/min. In 5 of them transient unstable fibrillation was observed immediately before conversion to a stable sinus rhythm. In one patient the atrial flutter was not influenced by atrial stimulation.

In our patients, in contrast to premature stimuli given high in the right atrium, premature stimuli given low in the right atrium during atrial flutter did markedly influence the time relations of the tachycardia. Pacemaker reset took place in all patients studied.

Our results are not compatible with the theory that atrial flutter in man is caused by a circus movement involving a large part of the atrium. They are in agreement with either an unprotected focus located low in the atrium or a reciprocal rhythm situated in a small area low in the atrium or the upper part of the A-V node.

In the latter situation longitudinal dissociation of the upper part of the A-V node must be present (103, 124). The circuit of such a reciprocal rhythm could consist of antegrade conduction through the upper part of the A-V node by pathway α, retrograde conduction through the upper part of the A-V node by pathway β, and small piece of atrium connecting pathways β and α.

SUMMARY

The two most favoured theories on the mechanism of atrial flutter in man are: a circus movement or a rapidly firing ectopic focus. Based on the assumption that a circus movement involving a large part of the atrium would react differently to an atrial premature beat than a rapidly firing ectopic focus, we studied the response to electrically induced atrial premature beats given high and low on the atrium.

Our results are compatible with either an unprotected ectopic focus located low in the atrium, or a reciprocal rhythm situated in a very small area low in the atrium or upper part of the A-V node, as responsible for the atrial flutter in our six patients.

CHAPTER 5

A-V JUNCTIONAL TACHYCARDIAS

The exact site and mechanism of impulse formation in patients with A-V junctional tachycardias is still largely unknown.

We wondered whether the response to electrically induced premature beats in patients with A-V junctional tachycardias could shed some light on this problem. Seven patients in which prior to the stimulation studies a diagnosis of A-V junctional tachycardia was made, were studied.

In four of these patients we also studied the initiation of their tachycardias.

CRITERIA

Patients were accepted for this study if their conventional and intra-atrial electrocardiograms fulfilled the following criteria:

1. Similar QRS complexes during tachycardia and sinus rhythm.
2. An 1 to 1 relation between ventricular and atrial activation.
3. A ventricular rate between 115 and 220/minute.
4. Activation during the tachycardia of the atria in a caudocranial direction, as recorded from intra-atrial leads.
5. During sinus rhythm a PR interval of 0.14 sec or more without signs of pre-excitation.

TABLE 3

Patient	Sex	Age	Frequency of attacks	Time period
A	male	47	first attack	
B	male	10	4 to 9 a year	5 years
C	female	61	about 5 a year	30 years
D	female	56	about 5 a year	10 years
E	male	62	last year almost continuously	20 years
F	female	63	3 to 4 times a week	2 years
G	female	23	last year almost continuously	5 years

It is clear that these criteria do not exclude tachycardias originating low in the atrium. Table 3 gives the sex, age, frequency of attacks and the time period of the seven patients studied.

Table 4 lists the frequencies of these tachycardias and the distances, both between the beginning of the QRS complex and the beginning of the Pwave (Q-P interval) and between the beginning of the Pwave and the QRS complex (P-Q interval). These measurements were made from intra-atrial leads.

TABLE 4

Patient	Frequency	Q-P interval	P-Q interval
A	210/min	60 msec	220 msec
B	220/min	130 msec	150 msec
C	220/min	160 msec	120 msec
D	165/min	50 msec	310 msec
E	165/min	200 msec	160 msec
F	115/min	50 msec	460 msec
G	140/min	215 msec	230 msec

From table 4 it becomes clear that in four of our patients the P wave was halfway between two QRS complexes. In the other three patients (A, D and F) the P wave followed shortly upon the preceding QRS complex.

All patients entered the catheterization room with a tachycardia. In the first three patients the study was stopped at the time the tachycardia was terminated. In the other four patients we also studied the way tachycardias could be initiated. We followed the protocol outlined in chapter 3.

1. *Identification of atrial rhythm, its relation with ventricular rhythm and if possible the direction of atrial activation*

As said before, all patients showed atrial activation in a caudocranial direction and a 1 to 1 relation between ventricular and atrial rhythm. The ventricular frequency ranged from 115/min to 220/min.

2. *The influence of one, or if possible two, induced atrial premature beats on the time relations of the tachycardia*

In three of our patients (A, B, and C) a single atrial premature beat given untill the refractory period of the atrium was reached, did not influence the

arrhythmia. The atrial premature beats were followed by a fully compensatory pause. No influence of the induced atrial beats on the ventricular
rhythm was noted. (An example is given in figure 15).

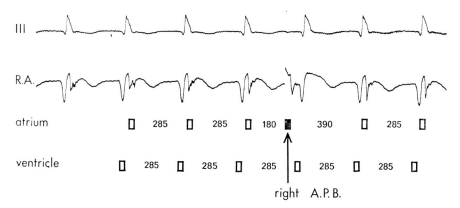

Fig. 15. Patient A. A right atrial premature beat given after an interval of 180 msec
is followed by a fully compensatory pause at the atrial level. No influence is seen
on the ventricular rhythm.

In patients D (fig. 16) and F, the induced atrial premature beats, given up
to the refractory period of the right atrium were followed by a QRS complex occurring after the same R-R interval as the tachycardia cycle.

The next QRS complex of the tachycardia however, occurred after an
interventricular interval shorter than the tachycardia R-R interval (see
fig. 17). As far as we know, this finding has been reported before only once
by Katz and Pick (60) (page 339, fig. 188). They considered this an example
of concealed A-V conduction. The atrial impulse penetrates the A-V junction but fails to reach the ventricles. In passing the A-V junction this impulse
reaches the ectopic pacemaker in the A-V node, discharges it and changes
its 'time table'. Thereafter the tachycardia resumes at the original cyclelength.
In our opinion a much likelier explanation can be given if one holds a
reciprocal mechanism responsible for the tachycardia in these patients
(fig. 18).

In patients A, B, C and D the tachycardia could not be terminated by a
single atrial premature beat.

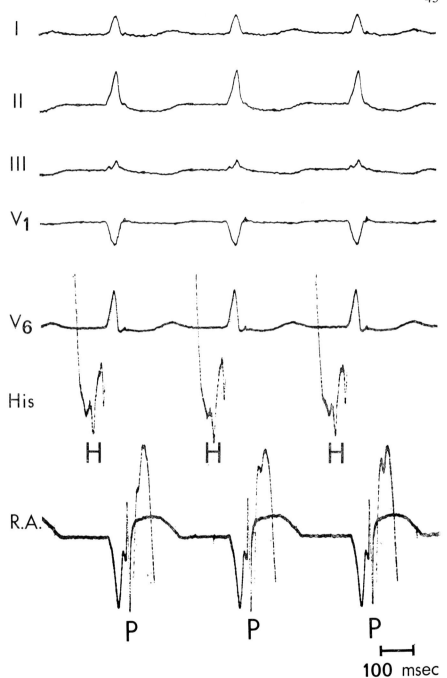

Fig. 16. Patient D. Simultaneous registration of lead I, II, III, V$_1$, V$_6$, His bundle and right atrium during an A-V junctional tachycardia. It can be seen that the QRS complex is preceded by a His bundle complex (H-V interval: 30 msec) and that the QRS complex is followed by the P wave after an interval of 50 msec.

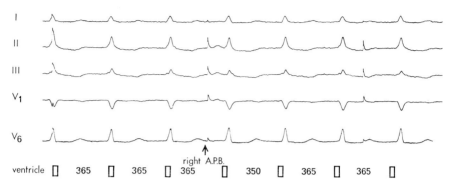

Fig. 17. Patient D. A right atrial premature beat given after an interval of 185 msec does not result in earlier appearance of the QRS complex immediately following this premature beat, but shortens the next R-R interval. See figure 18 for the explanation of this phenomenon.

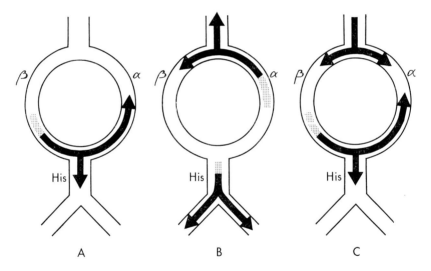

Fig. 18. Possible explanation for the findings shown in fig. 17. The tachycardia is assumed to be the result of an impulse circulating in a reciprocal pathway in the A-V junction. As shown in figures A and B ventricular activation precedes atrial activation. An appropriately timed atrial premature beat enters the reciprocal circuit at its atrial end and preexcites pathway β. This results in ventricular activation at an earlier time than expected during the tachycardia (C).

In patient E an early premature beat was followed by a slightly less than compensatory interval (fig. 19). On further shortening of the premature beat interval the tachycardia was terminated (fig. 20).

In patient F an early right atrial premature beat given after an interval of 225 msec ended the tachycardia (fig. 21).

Patient G: During the tachycardia (fig. 22 and 23) the interval between two atrial or two ventricular complexes measured 430-465 msec. Figure 24

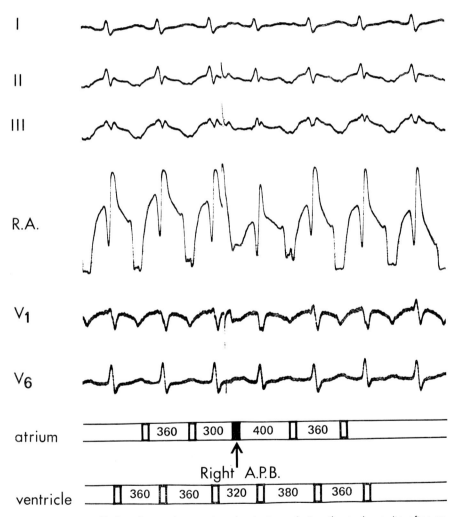

Fig. 19. Patient E. A right atrial premature beat given during the tachycardia after an interval of 300 msec captures the ventricle. The interval between the premature beat and the next atrial complex is slightly less than compensatory.

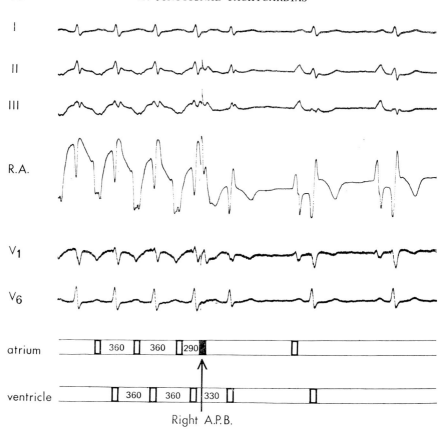

Fig. 20. Patient E. A right atrial premature beat given during the tachycardia after an interval of 290 msec terminates the tachycardia.

shows what happened following the induction of right atrial premature beats. On shortening the premature beat interval from 425 to 310 msec, no influence was noted on the ventricular rhythm, the interval from the premature atrial beat to the next atrial complex (A-A$_1$ interval) was fully compensatory. On further shortening the premature beat interval from 310 to 185 msec the ventricular complex (V$_1$) following the premature atrial beat occurred at a shorter interval than during the tachycardia, indicating ventricular capture by the premature atrial beat. At a premature beat interval of 185 msec this interval (V-V$_1$) measured 380 msec, the interval between V$_1$ and the next tachycardia complex being less than compensatory. (This is shown at greater magnification in figure 25). The refractory period of the right

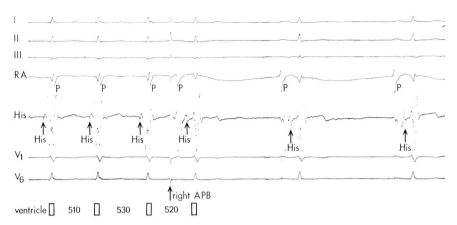

Fig. 21. Patient F. A right atrial premature beat given after an interval of 225 msec terminates the tachycardia.

atrium was reached at a premature beat interval of 165 msec. At premature beat intervals of less than 185 msec however, V_1 - V_2 became somewhat longer again because of lengthening of the interval between stimulus artefact and subsequent atrial activation.

It was never possible to terminate the tachycardia by a single premature atrial beat.

The question arises why one could shorten the atrial premature beat interval during the tachycardia from 425 to 310 msec before any shortening of the V - V_1 interval became manifest.

This is easy to understand if one realizes that stimulation was done high in the right atrium. As can be seen in figure 23 the time necessary for the impulse to travel from close to the tricuspid valve ring to the right atrial superior caval vein junction was approximately 115 msec. So it is likely that it will take about the same time before a stimulus given high in the right atrium reaches the A-V node.

3. The influence of one, if possible two, induced ventricular premature beats on the time relations of the tachycardia

This could only be systematically studied in patients C, D, E, F and G. In patients A and B, on advancing the electrode catheter into the right ventricle, two mechanically induced ventricular premature beats terminated the tachycardia.

48

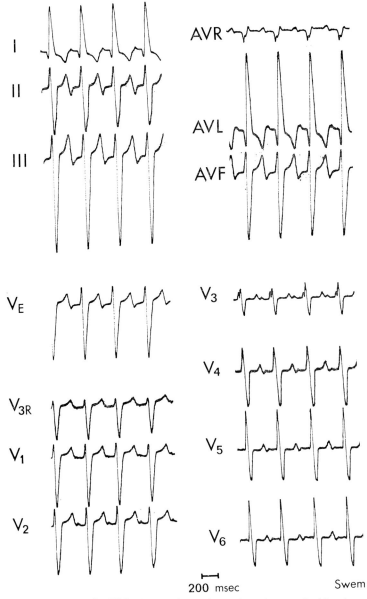

Fig. 22. Patient G. ECG during the tachycardia, showing highly abnormal QRS complexes (the patient suffered from a cardiomyopathy). The P waves are sandwiched in between the QRS complexes. They are negative in lead II, III and AVF. The QRS complexes were similar during tachycardia and sinus rhytrm.

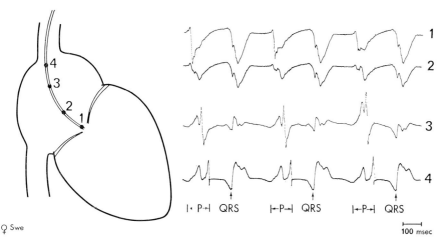

Fig. 23. Patient G. Simultaneous recording during the tachycardia from four intra-atrial leads. It is clearly shown that:
1. atrial activation is in a caudo-cranial direction
2. the P wave measures 115 msec.

In patient E both one and two induced right ventricular premature beats were followed by a fully compensatory interval before the next QRS complex of the tachycardia occurred (an example is given in figure 26).

In patient C one early ventricular premature beat was followed by a tachcardia QRS complex at slightly less than a fully compensatory interval (fig. 27). Two successive ventricular premature beats terminated the tachycardia (fig. 28).

In patient D a ventricular premature beat after an interval of 190 msec (cycle length of the tachycardia 365 msec) was followed by a less than fully compensatory interval (fig. 29). One ventricular premature beat given after an interval of 180 msec terminated the tachycardia (see fig. 30).

The same phenomena were observed in patient F (see fig. 31). In patient G a ventricular premature beat (V_1) given after an interval of 360 msec or less was followed by a less than compensatory interventricular interval (fig. 32). On shortening the premature beat interval ($V - V_1$) the distance between the induced ventricular beat (V_1) and the retrograde activation of the atrium (A_1) increased. This indicates that retrograde conduction through the A-V node became increasingly hampered (see fig. 33). At a premature beat interval of 290 msec retrograde conduction was blocked, resulting in termination of the tachycardia (fig. 34). The pause following thereafter was ended by a sinus escape beat.

50

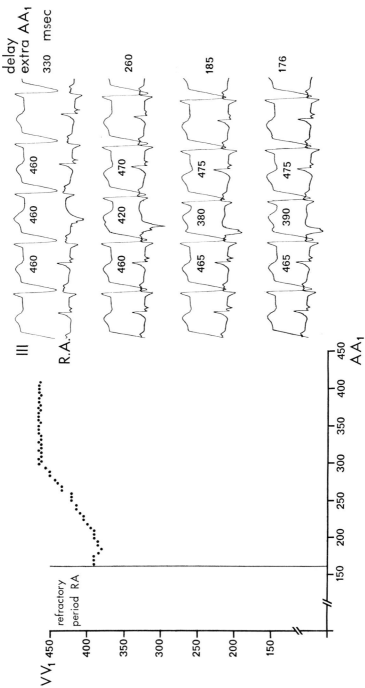

Fig. 24. Patient G. The influence of a single electrically induced right atrial premature beat on an A-V junctional tachycardia. Gradual shortening of the premature beat interval (A-A$_1$ interval) below an interval of 310 msec results in earlier appearance of ventricular activation (V$_1$). The right atrium becomes refractory to stimulation at an A-A$_1$ interval of 165 msec.

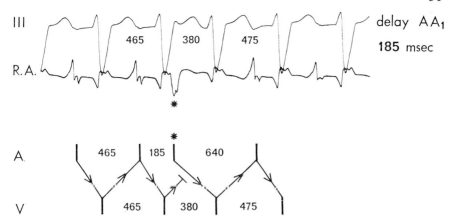

Fig. 25. Patient G. At an A-A$_1$ interval of 185 msec the V-V$_1$ interval measures 380 msec. It is clear that the interval between V$_1$ and the next tachycardia complex is less than fully compensatory.

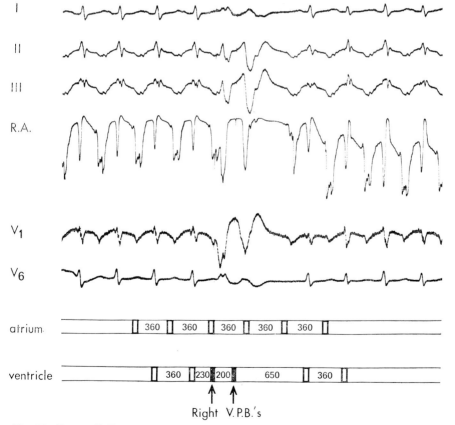

Fig. 26. Patient E. Two electrically induced early right ventricular premature beats do not influence the time relations of the tachycardia.

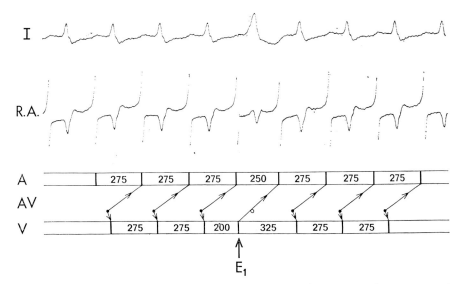

Fig. 27. Patient C. A single right ventricular premature beat given after an interval of 200 msec is followed by the next tachycardia QRS complex at a slightly less than fully compensatory interval.

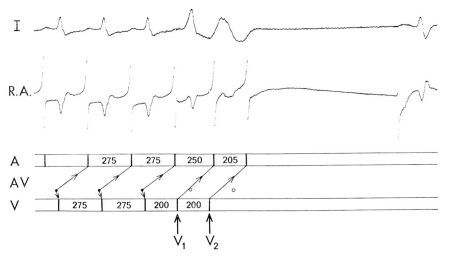

Fig. 28. Patient C. Termination of tachycardia by two consecutive right ventricular premature beats. As shown in the diagram both premature beats pass the A-V junction before the expected occurrence of the tachycardia impulse (represented here by open circles).

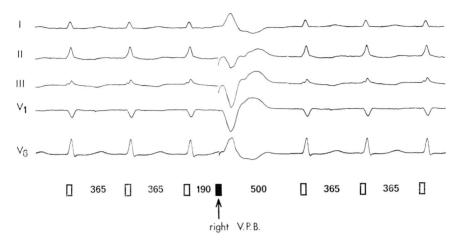

Fig. 29. Patient D. A single right ventricular premature beat given after an interval of 190 msec is followed during the tachycardia by a less than fully compensatory pause.

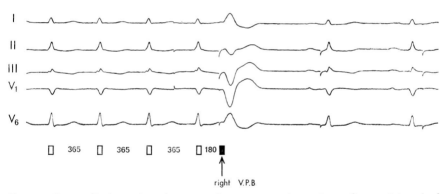

Fig. 30. Patient D. A single right ventricular premature beat given after an interval of 180 msec terminates the tachycardia.

4. *The result of driving the atrium at rates above the tachycardia frequency*

This was only done in patient G. In this patient driving the right atrium at rates above the tachycardia frequency resulted in 1 to 1 A-V conduction up to driving frequencies of 175/min. Thereafter Wenckenbach type of second degree A-V block developed. Figure 35 shows, as soon as driving the atrium at a frequency of 155/min. was discontinued, the ventricular complex resulting from the last atrial stimulus was followed by a retrograde P wave,

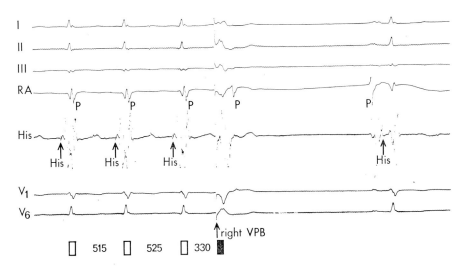

Fig. 31. Patient F. A single right ventricular premature beat given after an interval of 330 msec terminates the tachycardia.

immediately initiating again the tachycardia at its original frequency. Driving the atrium at frequencies between 400/min and 500/min led to atrial fibrillation.

These electrically induced periods of atrial fibrillation were shortlived, lasting maximally up to 4 minutes. The pause following these episodes was terminated by a sinus escape. The subsequent ventricular complex was always followed by retrograde atrial activation, initiating a new tachycardia.

In patient G we also drove the right ventricle at rates above the tachycardia frequency. 1 to 1 retrograde conduction was seen up to a driving rate of 160/min.

As shown in figure 36 when driving was discontinued the retrogradely conducted P wave was always immediately followed by the well-known tachycardia.

When driving was done at rates above 160/min. a Wenckebach type of ventriculo-atrial conduction resulted. Figure 37 shows how discontinuation of driving at the time when retrograde conduction to the atrium was blocked, resulted in a pause terminated by a sinus beat. The QRS complex resulting from this sinus escape was followed by retrograde atrial activation, initiating a new tachycardia.

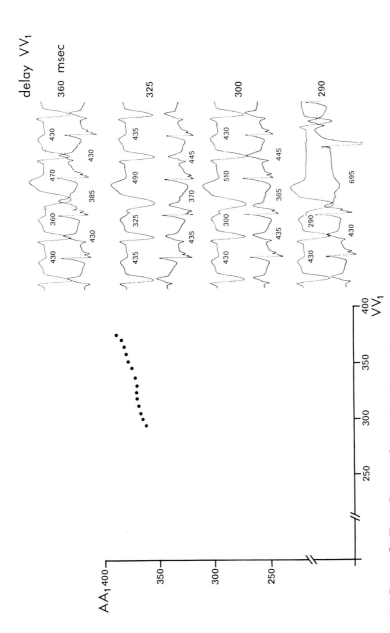

Fig. 32. Patient G. The influence of a single electrically induced right ventricular premature beat on the A-V junctional tachycardia. A ventricular premature beat (V_1) given after an interval of 360 msec or less is followed by a less than fully compensatory interventricular interval. Ventriculo-atrial conduction time increases on shortening the V-V_1 interval.

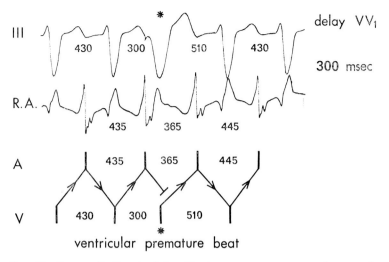

Fig. 33. Patient G. Detail of fig. 32 shown at greater magnification. A ventricular premature beat (V_1) given after an interval of 300 msec is followed by a less than compensatory interval.

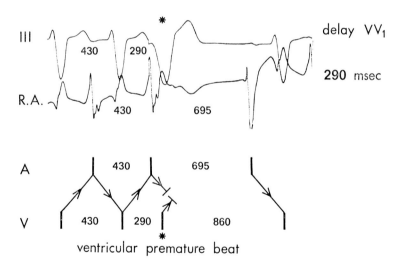

Fig. 34. Patient G. Detail of fig. 32 shown at greater magnification. A ventricular premature beat given after an interval of 290 msec terminates the tachycardia. As shown in the diagram this is caused by blockage of ventriculo-atrial conduction at this premature beat interval.

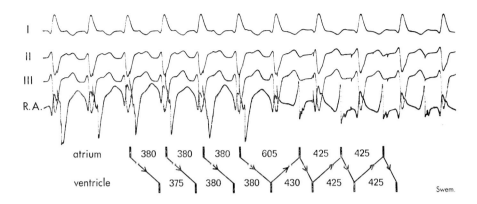

Fig. 35. Patient G. Driving the right atrium during the tachycardia at 155/min. results in atrial capture with 1 to 1 conduction to the ventricle. When atrial driving stops, the ventricular complex resulting from the last atrial stimulus is followed by a retrograde P wave immediately initiating again the tachycardia at its original frequency.

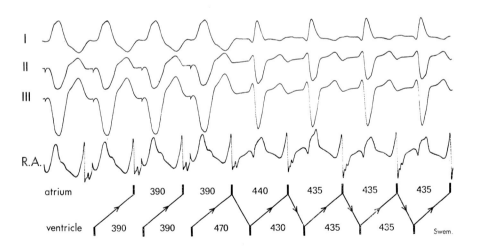

Fig. 36. Patient G. See text.

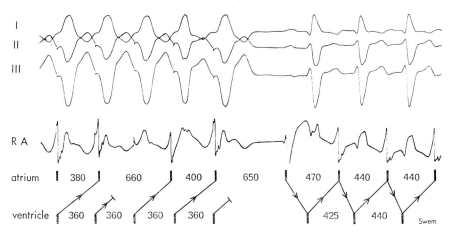

Fig. 37. Patient G. Termination of tachycardia by driving the right ventricle at rates above the tachycardia frequency. The mechanism is discussed in the text.

INITIATION OF TACHYCARDIAS

In patients A, B and C the study was ended when the tachycardia was successfully terminated.

In patients D, E and F the way tachycardias could be initiated was systematically studied by inducing premature beats during driving the right atrium and right ventricle.

In patient G every time the tachycardia was terminated (either by one ventricular premature beat, or overdriving from right atrium or right ventricle) the sinus escape that ended the post-tachycardia pause was immediately followed by retrograde atrial activation, and a new tachycardia.

a. Induction of one or two atrial premature beats during regular driving of the right atrium

In patient D during regular driving of the right atrium with a cycle length of 600 msec a single atrial premature beat given after an interval of 300 msec initiated a tachycardia.

As can be seen in figure 38 this atrial premature beat is followed after 410 msec by a QRS complex. This QRS complex is followed by the tachycardia.

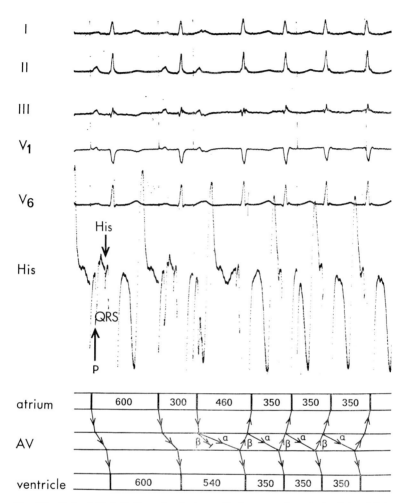

Fig. 38. Patient D. Initiation of a tachycardia by way of a single right atrial premature beat. During regular driving of the right atrium (BCL 600 msec) a right atrial premature beat (premature beat interval 300 msec) is followed by a tachycardia. The interval between the ventricular complex of the driven rhythm and the first ventricular complex of the tachycardia measures 540 msec. The length of this interval makes an A V junctional escape beat as the initiating mechanism for the tachycardia very unlikely. As shown in the diagram the initiation of the tachycardia can easily be explained if one assumes the presence of longitudinal dissociation in the A-V junction.

Similar observations were made in patient F. A single right atrial premature beat given after 400 msec during regular driving of the right atrium with a cycle length of 750 msec, reproducibly initiated a tachycardia (fig. 39).

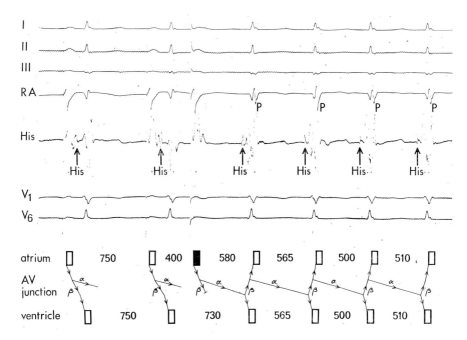

Fig. 39. Patient F. Iinitiation of a tachycardia by way of a single right atrial premature beat, given after 400 msec, during regular driving of the right atrium with a cycle length of 750 msec. A similar mechanism is assumed as in patient D.

In patient E an atrial premature beat, given after an interval of 320 msec during regular driving of the right atrium with a basic cycle length of 610 msec, reproducibly initiated a tachycardia. As shown in figure 40 the QRS complex resulting from the induced premature beat is followed after 200 msec by a P wave, clearly negative in lead II and III. This P wave indicating atrial activation in a caudo-cranial direction is followed by a tachycardia. In patient G the spontaneous recurrences of the tachycardia, after manoeuvres that ended the tachycardia, show that the QRS complex after the sinus escape is always followed by a P wave negative in lead II, III and AVF. This sequence (sinus P-QRS-retrograde P) is followed by the tachycardia.

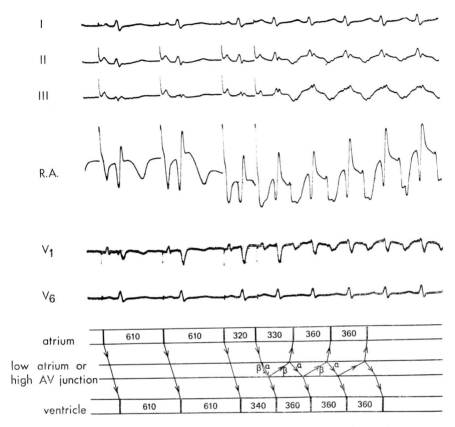

Fig. 40. Patient E. Initiation of a tachycardia by way of a single right atrial premature beat, given after an interval of 320 msec, during regular driving of the right atrium (basic cycle length 610 msec). The premature beat is conducted to the ventricles. This QRS complex is followed by a P wave negative in lead II and III. Thereafter a tachycardia is present. The presence of two pathways with different properties can explain the mechanism of initiation of this tachycardia.

b. Induction of one or two ventricular premature beats during regular driving of the right ventricle

In patient D and F shortening the premature beat interval of a single ventricular premature beat during right ventricular driving resulted in retrograde conduction towards the atrium till the right ventricle became refractory to stimulation. No tachycardia could be initiated in this way. The effect of two consecutive ventricular premature beats during regular driving of the right ventricle was not studied.

In patient E it was possible to induce a tachycardia with help of a single ventricular premature beat.

When during regular driving of the right ventricle with a basic cycle length of 610 msec, a ventricular premature beat was given after an interval of 280 msec, retrograde conduction towards the atrium was seen. This complex was followed after 330 msec by a negative P wave in lead II and III. This negative P wave was followed after 170 msec by the first QRS complex of the tachycardia. This sequence is shown in figure 41.

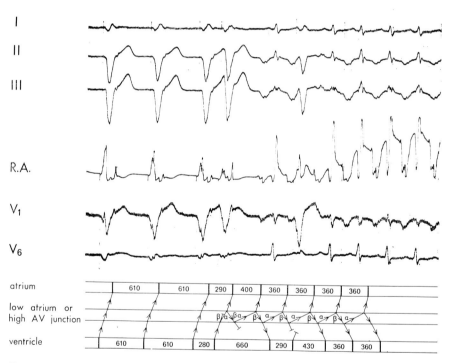

Fig. 41. Patient E. Initiation of a tachycardia by way of a single right ventricular premature beat. When during regular driving of the right ventricle (basic cycle length 610 msec) a right ventricular premature beat is induced after an interval of 280 msec retrograde conduction to the atrium is seen. This atrial complex is followed after 330 msec by a P wave negative in lead II and III. This is followed by the tachycardia. The diagram shows how the initiation of the tachycardia can be explained by assuming a reciprocal mechanism.

In patient G an analysis of initiation of tachycardias by ventricular premature beats could not be done, since every retrograde P following an electrically induced ventricular premature beat was immediately followed by a tachycardia.

DISCUSSION

A-V junctional tachycardias have been classified according to their character (paroxysmal vs non-paroxysmal), their site of origin (high, middle and low in the A-V junction) and their mechanism (focal vs reciprocal).

Pick and Dominguez (111) divided the 'active' A-V nodal tachycardias in two types. The first, which they called non-paroxysmal A-V nodal tachycardia, shows only a moderately increased discharge rate (70/min to 130/min) and lacks the sudden onset and abrupt termination characteristic for the second type called paroxysmal A-V nodal tachycardia. The frequency of the second type ranges between 150/min to 220/min.

The paroxysmal type was found as a rule in patients free from demonstrable cardiovascular abnormalities. This was the exception for the non-paroxysmal type where it was found primarily after digitalis excess, intracardiac surgery, coronary artery disease with or without myocardial infarction, and myocarditis.

The non-paroxysmal type is frequently associated with complete retrograde A-V block and a minor degree of antegrade A-V block, permitting capture of some impulses of the atrial pacemaker. All our seven patients had a tachycardia of the paroxysmal form. Patient F showed during her tachycardia a ventricular rate of only 115/min. The sudden onset and abrupt termination of the tachycardia however made us decide to accept this as a paroxysmal A-V junctional tachycardia. In two of our patients (A and D) the tachycardias became manifest after the onset of their angina pectoris, which suggests that in these patients, contrary to the common belief, the tachycardias might have been related to coronary artery disease. Patient F, who was referred to our department by Dr. J. Verheij, Dijkzigtziekenhuis, Rotterdam, suffered from a non-obstructive cardiomyopathy. She was incapacitated by long lasting attacks of tachycardia and was admitted with severe congestive heart failure. We did not study patients fulfilling the criteria of a non-paroxysmal A-V nodal tachycardia.

According to the relation between the QRS complex and the P wave (negative in lead II, III and AVF) A-V junctional tachycardias have been divided, as far as their origin is concerned, into 'upper, middle and lower' nodal tachycardias.

Such a classification has been correctly criticized:

1. Frequently the beginning of the tachycardia is not registered and one does not know whether the P wave actually precedes or follows the first QRS complex of the tachycardia.

2. The relationship between QRS complex and P wave following A-V nodal discharge depends upon the time necessary for the A-V junctional impulse to travel in forward (towards the ventricle) and retrograde (towards the atrium) direction. For instance an electrocardiogram showing a QRS complex followed after 50 msec by a negative P wave in lead II and III can result from an A-V junctional impulse originating low in the A-V node, but also from a focus high in the A-V node with slow retrograde conduction towards the atrium.

In animal hearts it has been demonstrated that various types of nodal rhythm may originate in the atrio-nodal (AN) region, the Nodal-His (NH) region and the His bundle (Paes de Carvalho and Almeida (108), Hoffman and Cranefield (52), Watanabe and Dreifus (143)). The introduction of the systematic recording of potentials from the specific conduction system (Scherlag et al. (129)) seems promising for the location of impulse formation in the A-V junction and His bundle of the human heart, especially when combined with selective stimulation of different parts of the conduction system (Narula et al. (106)). As far as origin and mechanism of A-V junctional tachycardias are concerned, the two theories advanced are:
- a focal origin
- a reciprocal rhythm.
(see also chapter 2).
Examples of the first theory have been described by Scherf et al. (126). They assume that (to quote from their article) 'a premature beat arriving at the A-V nodal centers early in diastole may precipitate a rapid firing of impulses at this area. The A-V node, with its known inherent high degree of automatically, is triggered, under these circumstances, to send out of burst of discharges.'

This explanation has been critized. It is very unusual indeed to induce a regular, long-lasting atrial or ventricular tachycardia by one single stimulus, unless the patient is digitalized or the stimulus strength many times threshold and the stimulus duration longer than 2 msec.

The second possibility, a reciprocal mechanism, has received most followers. The proposed structure of the A-V junction, (Hoffman (53)) and the experimental evidence provided by Scherf and Shookhoff (124), Moe and Mendez (103) and Watanabe and Dreifus (143) point to the feasibility of such a mechanism in A-V junctional tachycardias. Studies from our department on A-V junctional properties in the human heart support this hypothesis (Durrer et al. (33), Schuilenburg and Durrer (131, 132)).

The way by which an atrial or a ventricular premature beat can initiate such a tachycardia is illustrated in figures 38, 39, 40 and 41. As shown in figures 3 and 4 since they are caused by identical mechanisms, atrial and ventricular echo beats are a frequent finding in patients with reciprocal A-V junctional tachycardias.

Recently Gettes and Yoshonis (40) enumerated six criteria for the diagnosis of reciprocating tachycardias; based upon observations on clinical electrocardiograms:

1. Lengthening of the P-R or R-P interval at the onset of the tachycardia.
2. A difference in configuration between the P wave initiating the tachycardia and the P waves recorded during the tachycardia.
3. The presence of retrograde P waves having the same configuration as the P waves recorded during the tachycardia.
4. The presence of atrial or ventricular echoes.
5. The resetting of the tachycardia by a ventricular ectopic beat.
6. The termination of the tachycardia with both a retrograde P wave and with a QRS complex.

I completely agree with points 2, 3, 4 and 6, but would like to comment upon the other two points.

Ad 1

In a clinical tracing where the site of the tachycardia initiating atrial premature beat is unknown, the demand that the P-R interval of this atrial premature beat should be longer than the one following a sinus beat is an unrealistic one.

If the atrial premature beat originates close to the A-V junction there can be marked slowing of the impulse permitting longitudinal dissociation in the A-V junction without the P-R interval becoming longer than that of the P-R interval of the preceding sinus beat. The rule is true however during driving of the atrium. The atrial premature beat that initiated a tachycardia in our patients during regular driving of the atrium always showed a longer P-R interval than that of the complexes of the regular driven basic rhythm.

The same observation was made by Coumel et al. (23) during their studies on initiation of A-V junctional reciprocal tachycardias.

Ad 5

In the differentiation between focal and reciprocal A-V junctional tachycardias, both Wenckebach and Winterberg (149) and Scherf et al. (126) pointed to the importance of atrial and ventricular extrasystoles. If these during the tachycardia are followed by a compensatory interval a reciprocal tachycardia would be impossible. If one wants to use this criterion in a fair way however, one has to induce atrial and ventricular premature beats during the tachycardia in a systematic way, up to the refractory period of atrium and ventricle. Even then it will not always be possible to reach the site of A-V junctional impulse formation prior to the moment of discharge of the next tachycardia impulse.

This will depend upon:

1. The distance between the site of origin of the atrial or ventricular premature beat and the site of origin of the tachycardia in the A-V junction.
2. The conduction properties of the A-V junctional tissue surrounding the site of origin of the tachycardia.
3. The frequency of the tachycardia and its resulting refractory period.

A fully compensatory pause following an atrial or ventricular beat during the tachycardia, therefore does not exclude a reciprocal mechanism. See also chapter 2.

In three of our patients (A, B and C) the induced atrial premature beats given during the tachycardia up to the refractory period of the right atrium did not influence the arrhythmia.

In none of these patients the tachycardia could be terminated by a single premature atrial beat.

A different response was seen in these patients following ventricular premature beats. In patient C, where ventricular premature beats could be induced systematically, a less than compensatory interval following the premature beat was seen. Two consecutive ventricular premature beats terminated the tachycardia. In patients A and B two mechanically induced ventricular premature beats (on advancing the catheter into the right ventricle) terminated the tachycardia.

These findings reveal that the tachycardia in patients A, B and C could be influenced and terminated from the ventricular end of the A-V junction. The behaviour following the very early ventricular premature beats (a less than compensatory interval) is in agreement with both a reciprocal mechanism and an unprotected focus. The termination of the tachycardias by one or two ventricular premature beats can be explained by assuming that these premature beats make the lower part of the reciprocal pathway refractory. The latter finding suggest a long proximal common pathway and a reciprocal circuit, located close to the ventricle. As pointed out before, Pick, Langendorf and Katz (109) however have described cases of depression of cardiac pacemakers by a single premature impulse. Such a mechanism will obviously be enhanced when two premature stimuli are given. One could argue that this mechanism was responsible for the termination of the tachycardias in patients A, B and C.

In patients A, B and C the initiation of tachycardias was unfortunately not studied. Our results indicate that without this knowledge it is impossible to decide between a focal origin or a reciprocal mechanism as responsible for the tachycardias in patients A, B and C.

In patient D and F the tachycardia could be initiated by one premature atrial beat. In figure 38 and 39 it can be seen that the QRS complex following the induced atrial premature beat is followed after 50 msec. by a retrograde P wave. It is very likely that longitudinal dissociation of the A-V junction permitting the initiation of a reciprocal tachycardia is responsible for this phenomenon. An A-V junctional escape beat as the initiating mechanism for the tachycardia seems unlikely in view of the short escape interval (shorter than the basic cycle length of the regular driven atrial rhythm). Also the events during the tachycardia following an induced atrial and ventricular premature beat, and the termination of the tachycardia by a single ventricular premature beat favour a reciprocal mechanism.

In patient E the tachycardia could not be influenced from the ventricular side. A single atrial premature beat however was followed by a less than compensatory tachycardia interval and an earlier one did even terminate the tachycardia.

The mechanism of initiation suggests a reciprocal tachycardia located low in the atrium or upper part of the A-V junction. The first location is

favoured by the different configuration of the retrograde P waves following
right ventricular driving as compared to the P waves during the tachycardia
(fig. 41).

An example of a supraventricular tachycardia, initiated and terminated
by a single atrial stimulus was reported by Barold et al. (3). In view of the
configuration of the P waves they thought that a circus movement at the
atrial level was responsible for the tachycardia. In patient G the tachycardia
could be influenced both from the atrial and ventricular side. This finding
combined with the way tachycardias could be initiated and terminated and
its behaviour during driving at rates above the tachycardia frequency all
speak in favour of a reciprocal A-V junctional tachycardia.

Stimulation studies in patients with reciprocal A-V junctional tachycardias
have been reported by Coumel et al. (23), Goldreyer and Bigger (42) and
Zeft and Mc Gowan (157). Coumel et al. (23) described several patients
where they could initiate and interrupt tachycardias by appropriately timed
atrial and ventricular premature beats. They also showed that premature
atrial and ventricular beats were not always followed by a fully compensatory interval. These authors could completely control the tachycardias
in two of their patients by simultaneous stimulation of atrium and ventricle
(see also chapter 7).

In the case reported by Goldreyer and Bigger (42) ventricular stimulation
was not performed. A reciproval tachycardia originating low in the atrium
can therefore not be excluded. They did not comment upon the influence
of atrial premature beats on the cycle length of the tachycardia. Zeft and
Mc Gowan (156) terminated a junctional tachycardia by way of a single
right ventricular premature beat. They also noted that right ventricular
premature beats, given with slightly longer premature beat intervals did
influence the time relations of the tachycardia. The tachycardia in their
patient could not be interrupted by atrial stimulation.

SUMMARY

In seven patients who entered the catheterization room with a diagnosis of
A-V junctional tachycardia we registered the influence of electrically induced
right atrial and right ventricular premature beats upon the time relations of
the tachycardia. In all patients it was possible to terminate the tachycardia
by one or two induced premature beats. In four of our patients the initiation

of the tachycardias was studied as well. In these four patients the results favour a reciprocal mechanism as responsible for the tachycardia. In one of them a location of the reciprocal pathway low in the atrium seemed more likely than an A-V junctional one. In the remaining three patients, where the initiation of the tachycardia was not studied, no definite diagnosis as to a focal origin or a reciprocal mechanism of the tachycardia could be made.

Our results indicate, that in order to come to a correct conclusion about the mechanism, responsible for the tachycardia, both, initiation, termination and the influence of premature beats upon the time relations of the tachycardia should be studied.

CHAPTER 6

TACHYCARDIAS RELATED TO THE PRE-EXCITATION SYNDROME

In 1930 Wolff, Parkinson and White (153) described patients with electrocardiograms showing a short PR interval, a delta wave and a wide QRS complex.

Since then similar and variant forms of this electrocardiographic pattern have been described. (Burch and Kimball (11), Scherf and Cohen (127).

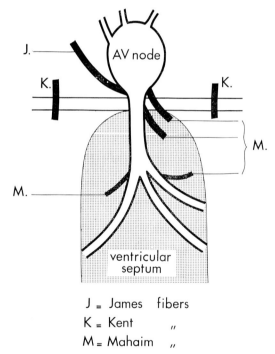

J = James fibers
K = Kent "
M = Mahaim "

Fig. 42. Schematic representation of the location of the anomalous A-V pathways playing a possible role in the pre-excitation syndrome.
J = James fibres; K = Kent fibres; M = Mahaim fibres.

Both the peculiar configuration of the electrocardiogram suggesting earlier than normal excitation of the whole or part of the ventricles following atrial activation, and the explanation of the frequently occurring tachycardias in these patients have been a problem for years.

As Durrer, Schuilenburg and Wellens (35) have recently outlined, new advances enable us to shed some light on this problem:

1. The availability of a comprehensible classification of the relation between the several possible abnormal anatomic connections between atria and ventricles or parts of the A-V conduction system and their resulting electrocardiographic patterns (Lev (76), Ferrer (38), see fig. 42, 43).
2. The introduction of electrical stimulation allowing the study of A-V conduction in the human heart and the study and treatment of conduction abnormalities and arrhythmias.
3. The possibility of recording epicardial activation during surgery in patients with pre-excitation (Durrer and Roos (30)).
4. The cure of life-threatening tachycardias and 'normalization' of the QRS complex by dividing the abnormal connection between atrium and ventricle in patients with the pre-excitation syndrome (Burchell et al. (13), Cobb et al. (18), and Boineau and Moore (5)).

This chapter reports the results obtained during electrical stimulation of the hearts of patients who showed electrocardiographic evidence of pre-excitation and had a history of tachycardias.

Eleven patients were studied (in table 5 they are tentatively classified according to their type of pre-excitation). Eight fulfilled the 'classic' Wolff-Parkinson-White (153) syndrome criteria:
– a PR interval of 0.12 sec. or less
– a delta wave
– a QRS width of 0.12 sec. or more.

Five of them belonged to type A, and three to type B, according to the classification of Rosenbaum et al. (118). One patient (I) showed a normal PR interval, a small delta wave and a QRS width of 0.10 sec. Two patients (J and K) showed a short PR interval (0.12 sec or less), no delta wave and a QRS width of 0.10 sec.

In all these patients the initiation and termination of their tachycardias was studied by way of electrically induced atrial and ventricular premature beats. Also the influence of induced premature beats on the time relations of the tachycardia was registered.

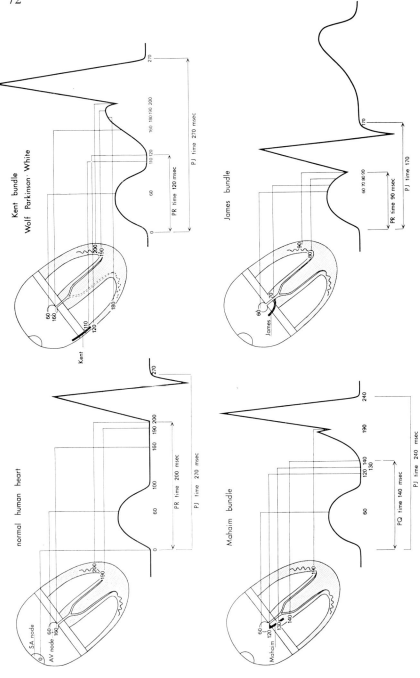

Fig. 43. Scheme showing the relation between excitation of the heart and the electrocardiogram as recorded in a standard lead, in a normal patient and in patients with a Kent bundle, a Mahaim bundle and a James bundle.

TABLE 5

Patient	Sex	Age	Type of pre-excitation	Frequency tachycardia	Frequency of attacks	Time period
A	male	20	W.P.W. type B	220/min.	twice a week	3 years
B	female	47	W.P.W. type B	170/min.	once a week	4 years
C	male	51	W.P.W. type B	205/min.	2-3 times a week	40 years
D	male	44	W.P.W. type A	180/min.	once a day	23 years
E	male	54	W.P.W. type A	140/min.	twice a year	18 years
F	female	46	W.P.W. type A	150/min.	almost daily during the last two years	28 years
G	male	51	W.P.W. type A	185/min.	2 times a week	4 years
H	female	24	W.P.W. type A	205/min.	2 times a week	10 years
I	male	8	Mahaim?	210/min.	2-3 times a year	5 years
J	female	38	James	250/min.	2 times in 4 years	4 years
K	female	35	James?	220/min.	6 times a year	18 years

'CLASSIC' WOLFF-PARKINSON-WHITE SYNDROME

The many theories advanced (see Scherf and Cohen (127)) for the explanation of the electrocardiographic patterns of the Wolff-Parkinson-White syndrome can essentially be divided into two groups:

a. a abnormal A-V bypass resulting in concomitant ventricular activation by way of the normal A-V conduction pathway and the abnormal A-V bypass (Kent bundle).
b. accelerated conduction through the A-V junction. A concept introduced by Prinzmetal et al. (116), recently reintroduced in a revised way by Sherf and James (133).

Much has been written to explain the mechanism of the frequently occurring tachycardias in these patients. Based upon observations on clinical electrocardiograms a circus movement involving antegrade conduction through the normal A-V conduction pathway and retrograde conduction through the abnormal A-V bypass was advanced as the pathway present during the tachycardia (Wolferth and Wood (152), Wolff and White (154) and Pick and Katz 110)). Durrer et al. (31) were the first to study this hypothesis systematically by inducing atrial and ventricular premature beats during sinus rhythm and regular driven atrial and ventricular rhythms.

It was demonstrated that in two patients with W.P.W. type B a supraventricular tachycardia could repeatedly be induced by right atrial and ventricular premature beats given so early that the functional properties of the normal and abnormal A-V conduction pathway became dissociated.

During regular atrial stimulation a very early atrial premature beat was found to be blocked in the accessory bundle (Kent bundle) but conducted slowly through the normal A-V conduction system. Following normal excitation of the ventricles this impulse was conducted retrogradely through the Kent bundle towards the atrium. This atrial activation descended down into the normal A-V conduction pathway again, thereby completing the first cycle of the ensuing tachycardia.

During ventricular driving a very early induced ventricular premature beat was conducted to the atrium by way of the Kent bundle while retrograde conduction through the A-V node was blocked. This retrograde atrial activation was followed by antegrade conduction through the recovered normal A-V conduction pathway, leading to normal excitation of the ventricle. This was followed by retrograde conduction towards the atrium using the Kent bundle. Again the impulse from the retrogradely activated atrium by descending down into the normal A-V conduction system completed the first cycle of the tachycardia.

These observations supported the hypothesis that during the tachycardia a circus movement involving the atrium, the normal A-V conduction pathway, the ventricles and the Kent bundle was present. A strong argument for such a mechanism was the finding that during the tachycardia in one patient with W.P.W. type B, electrically induced early atrial or ventricular premature beats resulted in shortening of one ventricular cycle, without changes in length of the following ventricular cycles (see fig. 13 and 16 from Durrer et al. (31)). Further shortening of the interval of the atrial or ventricular premature beats resulted in termination of the tachycardia by creating a refractory zone in the pathway of the circulating impulse.

On mapping the epicardial excitation during surgery for an atrial septal defect in a patient with W.P.W. type B, Durrer and Roos (30) had already found that the earliest point of excitation of the ventricule was situated on the high lateral aspect of the right ventricle close to the A-V sulcus. At this location epicardial excitation started 120 msec after the beginning of atrial activation from the sinus node. This observation was later confirmed by Burchell et al. (13), Cobb et al. (18), and Boineau and Moore (5).

The similar results of epicardial excitation mapping in patients with the W.P.W. syndrome type B indicate that the typical electrocardiogram in these patients can be the result of an accessory atrioventricular pathway inserting into the anterolateral aspect of the right ventricle. These observations coupled with the outcome of the electrical stimulation studies in our patients strongly suggested that a circus movement using the A-V nodal-His pathway and the accessory A-V pathway can be the mechanism for tachycardias in W.P.W. type B.

Such a circus movement can theoretically run in two directions:
1. with atrio – ventricular conduction via His' bundle and ventriculo – atrial conduction by way of the Kent bundle.
2. with atrio-ventricular conduction through the Kent bundle and ventriculo-atrial conduction through the His bundle.

The QRS complexes during the tachycardia will under those circumstances show:

1. Small QRS complexes (resulting from antegrade His conduction) or typical right or left bundle branch configuration (when one of the bundle branches is refractory during the tachycardia), and
2. wide QRS complexes with maximal pre-excitation configuration (resulting from antegrade Kent conduction).

It should be stressed that these two tachycardias do not necessarily have the same rate because their pathways are not identical.

It is very important to realize that not all of the tachycardias in patients with W.P.W. syndrome are caused by a circus movement, because these patients have at least the same chance as other patients to suffer from atrial tachycardias, atrial flutter, atrial fibrillation, A-V junctional tachycardias and focal ventricular tachycardias.

Definite proof that a circus movement can be responsible for life-threatening attacks of tachycardia was given by Burchell et al. (13), Cobb et al. (18), and Boineau and Moore (5), when they operated upon patients with W.P.W. type B and made an incision in the area where the Kent bundle was located after mapping epicardial excitation. Unfortunately the first group saw, after a short period of 'normalization' of the QRS complex, a recurrence of pre-excitation. Burchell et al. (13) thought that too small an incision, located only on the endocardial site of the right atrium with the impossibility to evaluate the result of the incision due to procaine infiltration of the area was responsible for their result.

The work of Cobb et al. (18) and Boineau and Moore (5) however, resulted in complete disappearance of both pre-excitation (as manifested in the ECG) and tachycardias.

Dreifus et al. (28) and Edmonds and coworkers (37) demonstrated the feasibility of interrupting the tachycardia pathway at another site by dissecting the A-V node. Their patients suffered from tachycardias in the presence of W.P.W. type A.

In view of the difficulties of accurately locating the anomalous A-V connection in these patients, they decided upon dissection of the A-V node.

Results of our stimulation studies in the 'classic' Wolff-Parkinson-White syndrome

W.P.W. type B

The results in two (A and B) of our three patients with W.P.W. type B have been reported before (Durrer et al. (31)).

In the third patient (C) tachycardias could be initiated by a single atrial and ventricular premature beat during regular driving of respectively right atrium and right ventricle.

The tachycardias could be terminated by one electrically induced right atrial and ventricular beat. In this patient a third way of initiating a tachycardia, namely by way of an atrial echo beat, was discovered. This is shown in figures 44 and 45.

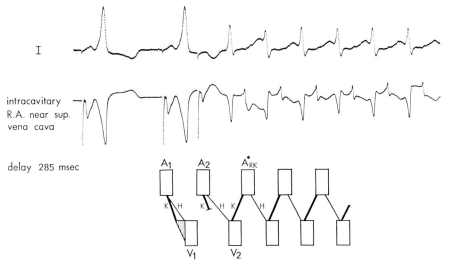

Fig. 44. Patient C. During regular driving of the right atrium (BLC 620 msec) an atrial premature beat given after an interval of 285 msec initiates a tachycardia. The configuration of the QRS complex following the atrial premature beat demonstrates the conduction to the ventricle by the His pathway only. Following ventricular activation, retrograde conduction to the atrium occurs by way of the Kent bundle. This atrial complex (A* RK) is able to activate the ventricle by way of the His pathway. This completes the first cycle of the tachycardia.

In patient C one premature atrial or ventricular beat induced during the tachycardia was followed by a fully compensatory pause. It was therefore not possible to change the time relations of the tachycardia by way of a single atrial or ventricular beat.

W.P.W. type A

As far as we know initation and termination of tachycardias in patients with W.P.W. type A have not been studied systematically. Also the influence of an induced single atrial or ventricular premature beat on the time relations

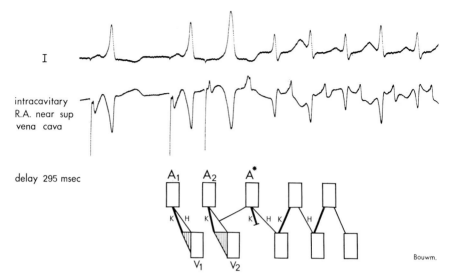

I

intracavitary
R.A. near sup
vena cava

delay 295 msec

Fig. 45. Patient C. A different mechanism of initiation of a tachycardia at an atrial premature beat interval of 295 msec (again the basic cycle length of the regular driven rhythm is 620 msec). The configuration of the QRS complex following the atrial premature beat shows that ventricular activation took place both by way of the Kent bundle and the His pathway. This QRS complex is followed by an atrial complex. The configuration of this P wave as recorded from the intra-atrial lead suggests that this is an atrial echo. This atrial complex finds the Kent bundle refractory and is conducted towards the ventricle by way of the His bundle only. Thereafter the tachycardia supervenes.

of the tachycardia in these patients is not known. Our results will therefore be reported in detail.

Initiation of tachycardias in Wolff-Parkinson-White syndrome type A

a. Right atrial stimulation

In patients D, E, F and H it was impossible to induce a tachycardia with a single right atrial premature beat during regular driving of the right atrium. In these four cases the right atrium became refractory to electrical stimulation before blockade of the impulse in either the Kent or His pathway occurred.

In patient G however during driving of the right atrium with a basic cycle length of 660 msec, an induced right atrial premature beat after an interval of 260 msec resulted in a tachycardia with QRS complexes measuring 135 msec in width and showing a configuration compatible with excitation of the ventricle by way of the Kent bundle only. The attacks of tachycardia were shortlived, measuring 8-16 beats and could readily be induced by right atrial premature beats up to a premature beat interval of 184 msec.

This represents the first reproducible demonstration of a circus movement with atrio-ventricular conduction through the Ken btundle and retrograde ventriculo-atrial conduction by way of the His' bundle (see fig. 46).

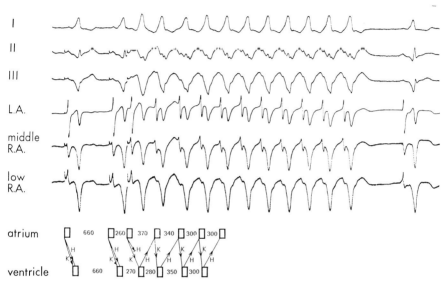

Fig. 46. Patient G. Initiation of a tachycardia. showing exclusive Kent conduction, by way of a single right atrial premature beat. The configuration of the QRS complex following a right atrial premature beat (premature beat interval 260 msec) during regular driving of the right atrium (BCL 660 msec) suggests conduction to the ventricle by way of the Kent bundle only. This QRS complex is followed by a tachycardia showing similar QRS complexes. As clarified in the diagram this could be a tachycardia with atrioventricular conduction through the Kent bundle and ventriculoatrial conduction through the His pathway.

The tachycardia always ended by a ventricular complex not being followed by an atrial complex (see fig. 46) indicating retrograde block of the His' bundle following that beat.

The observation that up to the refractory period of the right atrium (184 msec during driving with a basic cycle length of 670 msec) no appreciable delay in atrio-ventricular conduction through the Kent bundle is seen, clearly demonstrates a very important aspect of pre-excitation. In patients with very short refractory periods of their anomalous A-V connection the ventricles are a helpless victim if rapid supraventricular arrhythmias like atrial flutter or fibrillation occur. This indicates a possible mechanism of sudden death in patients with the preexcitation syndrome.

It illustrates the necessity of identifying those with such properties of their anomalous connection, and stresses the importance of further investigations to prevent these patients from fatal arrhythmias.

In patient F in which one atrial premature beat did not elicit a tachycardia two right atrial premature beats given in close succession resulted in a tachy-cardia. The shortening of the refractory period of the right atrium following the first premature beat made it possible to give such an early second premature beat that this impulse found the anomalous pathway towards the ventricle refractory. In this way a tachycardia with antegrade His conduction and retrograde Kent conduction could reproducibly be induced.

b. Left atrial stimulation

This was done in patient F, G and H. In our opinion it was not justified to perform a Ross catheterization only for the study of the mechanism of the tachycardias in patients with the preexcitation syndrome.

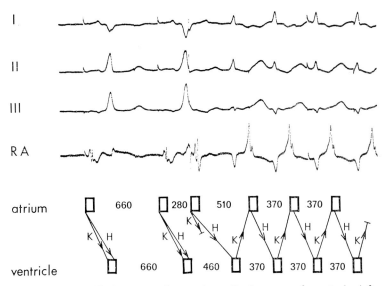

Fig. 47. Patient F. Initiation of a tachycardia by way of a single left atrial premature beat (premature beat interval 280 msec) during regular driving of the left atrium (BCL 660 msec). .

In patients F and H however the evaluation of co-existent mitral valve disease made such a procedure necessary. Patient G surprised us with an open foramen ovale.

In patient F a tachycardia could readily be induced by one premature left atrial beat given during regular left atrial driving (see fig. 47). This tachycardia showed antegrade His conduction.

In patient G on driving the left atrium with a basic cycle length of 660 msec., a left atrial premature beat given after an interval of 260 msec. initiated a tachycardia. The QRS complexes during the tachycardia were similar to the QRS complexes of the tachycardia that could be initiated from the right atrium in this patient (a tachycardia probably caused by a circus movement with antegrade Kent and retrograde His conduction) (See fig. 48).

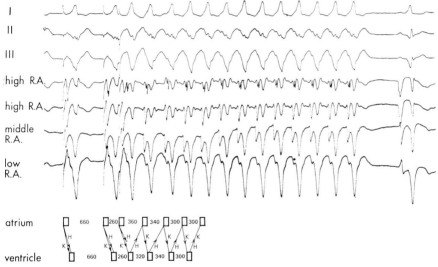

Fig. 48. Patient G. Initiation of a tachycardia, showing exclusive Kent conduction by way of a single left atrial premature beat. During regular driving of the left atrium (BCL 660 msec) a left atrial premature beat given after an interval of 260 msec initiates a tachycardia showing atrio-ventricular conduction by way of the Kent bundle only. Compare this figure with fig. 46; note the difference in QRS complex configuration during regular driving of the right and left atrium.

This tachycardia (measuring 8-17 beats) could be initiated reproducibly by one left atrial premature beat up to the refractory period of the left atrium. If one compares figure 46 and fgiure 48 it becomes clear that during driving of the right and left atrium with identical frequencies (basic cycle length of 660 msec.) the contribution to ventricular excitation by way of the anomalous connection is greater if stimulation is performed from the left atrium. This suggests that the atrial end of the abnormal A-V connection is situated on the left side.

In patient H one left atrial premature beat given during regular left atrial stimulation repeatedly resulted in a tachycardia with antegrade His and retrograde Kent conduction.

Electrically induced ventricular premature beats during regular driving of the ventricle

a. Right ventricular stimulation
In patient D shortening the interval of an induced right ventricular premature beat during regular driving of the right ventricle (basic cycle length 650 msec) resulted in a gradual increase in QP time. The P waves were repro-

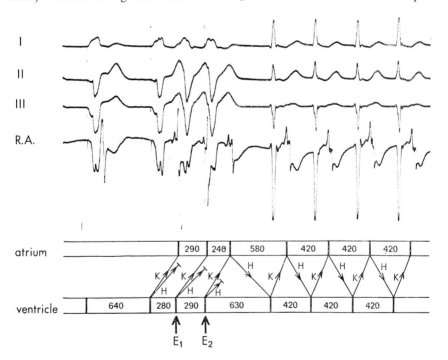

Fig. 49. Patient E. Initiation of a tachycardia by way of two right ventricular premature beats (E₁ and E₂) given in close succession. See text for discussion.

ducibly followed by a tachycardia with antregrade His conduction at a premature beat interval of 330 msec.

In patient E shortening the interval of the induced right ventricular premature beat resulted only in a slight increase in QP interval. The right ventricle became refractory to the premature stimulus without induction of a tachycardia. Two closely given right ventricular premature beats however resulted in a tachycardia. Depending upon the interval between these premature beats the mechanism responsible for the initation of the tachycardia was different.

(1) *Initiation of a tachycardia by way of the Kent bundle during blocked retrograde conduction through the His bundle.*

When the right ventricle was driven with a basic cycle length of 640 msec, two right ventricular premature beats were given after an interval of respectively 280 and 570 msec, following the last beat of the regular driven right ventricular rhythm.

The second ventricular premature beat was followed after 630 msec. by a small QRS complex initiating a tachycardia, showing antegrade His conduction (fig. 49).

From the work of Janse et al. (58) we know that a sudden increase in heart rate results in marked changes in refractoriness of the heart. These changes take several beats before becoming stable and are not identical in the conduction system and the ventricular muscular tissue. This may augment the dissociation in functional properties of the Kent and A-V node-His bundle pathway necessary for the initiation of the tachycardia by giving two premature beats instead of one. The second ventricular premature beat can be looked upon as the third beat of a tachycardia. Apparently, as shown in the diagram (see fig. 49), the first induced premature beat is followed by retrograde conduction towards the atrium by way of the Kent bundle and retrograde penetration far into the His-A-V junctional pathway. The second premature beat is again conducted retrogradely through the Kent bundle, but arrested at the ventricular end of the His bundle because this structure is now refractory.

As we know (31) this situation creates the possibility for the atrial impulse, which results from retrograde conduction through the Kent bundle, to enter the atrial end of the A-V junction and to return to the ventricles by way of the His bundle, thereby initiating a tachycardia.

(2) *Initiation of a tachycardia by way of a ventricular echo beat.* When during right ventricular driving two right ventricular premature beats were induced after an interval of respectively 350 and 590 msec. following the last beat of the regularly driven right ventricular rhythm, a different mode of initiation of the tachycardia was seen. As figure 50 demonstrates the second right ventricular premature beat was now followed, after 400 msec., by a smaller QRS complex measuring 90 msec. in width. After 580 msec. a small QRS complex is registered, initiating the tachycardia.

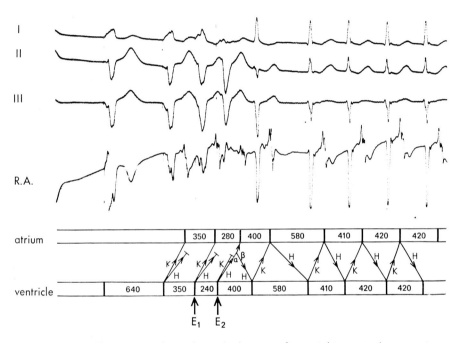

Fig. 50. Patient E. Initiation of a tachycardia by way of two right ventricular premature beats (E_1 and E_2) given in close succession. The mechanism is different from the one shown in fig. 49. As discussed in the text a ventricular echo beat as the initiating mechanism seems very likely.

In view of the short distance (400 msec.) between the second premature right ventricular beat and the first small QRS complex, and considering the distance between the first and the second of the smaller QRS complexes we feel that it is impossible to explain this sequence by the same mechanism as described under (1).

Using the longitudinal dissociation concept of the A-V node advanced by Scherf and Shookhoff (124) and Moe et al. (100) whereby the presence of two pathways (α and β) with different properties is assumed, it seems very likely that the first small QRS complex is a ventricular echo. Following the second right ventricular premature beat the A-V node is invaded from below. The impulse finds one pathway (α) refractory and travels by way of the other pathway (β). When the impulse arrives at the common pathway, it is propagated towards the atrium, but also back towards the ventricle by way of the now recovered α pathway. This impulse activates the ventricles and fulfils the criteria for a ventricular reciprocal beat or ventricular echo (Schuilenburg and Durrer (132)).

Atrial activation following the second ventricular premature beat and preceding the ventricular echo is probably the result of retrograde conduction by way of the Kent bundle only, the impulse being so delayed in the A-V node that it reaches the atrium when the atrium is refractory from the impulse resulting from retrograde Kent conduction. The configuration of the ventricular echo suggests that slightly aberrant conduction to the ventricles took place. The P wave following the echo beat is the result of retrograde conduction through the Kent bundle only, His' bundle being refractory. This impulse descends down towards the ventricles by way of the His bundle completing the first cycle of the ensuing tachycardia.

Patient F: for the same reason as in patient E it was not possible to initiate a tachycardia by way of one right ventricular premature beat. Two right ventricular premature beats however repeatedly resulted in a tachycardia, the mechanism being identical as mechanism I in patient E.

Patient G: In this patient a single early induced right ventricular premature beat was followed by a 'spontaneously occurring' second early right ventricular premature beat. Such a 'spontaneous' ventricular beat after an early electrically induced premature ventricular beat is in our experience not uncommon during electrical stimulation of the ventricle. They occur following stimulation close to the refractory period of the ventricle. The configuration of this beat is frequently similar to the electrically induced premature beat. We do not know whether they represent: (1) mechanically induced premature beats from the catheter point, (2) multiple firing following stimulation close to the refractory period or (3) re-entry by way of unindirectional block in closely adjacent Purkinje fibers followed by conduction through muscle tissue and re-entry into the Purkinje network at a distance (Hoffmann (53)). In view of the constant time relations between this 'spontaneous' ventricular premature beat to the foregoing ventricular premature beat and the low stimulusstrength the third explanation seems the most likely one.

The sequence of an induced early premature beat followed by a 'spontaneous' ventricular beat was repeatedly followed by a tachycardia. The explanation for the mechanism for initiation of the tachycardia is essentially the same as for patients E and F. It is important to note that in this patient (patient G), it was possible to initiate during atrial stimulation tachycardias with antegrade Kent and retrograde His conduction, while during ventricular stimulation (see fig. 51 during left ventricular stimulation) a tachycardia could be initiated that ran in the reversed direction. In both situations the His bundle was the A-V connection that was blocked on shortening the interval of the premature stimulus.

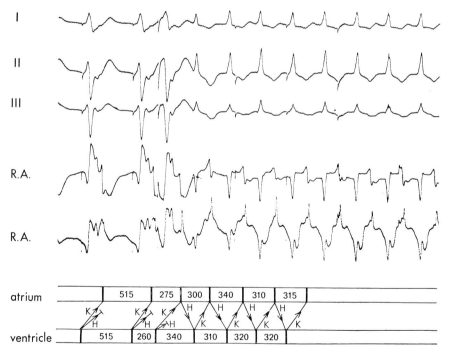

Fig. 51. Patient G. Initiation of a tachycardia by way of a single left ventricular premature beat. During regular driving of the left ventricle (BCL 515 msec) a premature beat was given after an interval of 260 msec. The possible mechanism of initiation of the tachycardia is shown in the diagram.

Patient H: no tachycardias could be initiated by one right ventricular premature beat, for reasons already given under patient E. Two right ventricular beats were not given.

b. Left ventricular stimulation

This was only done in patients F, G and H. In patients F and G one early left ventricular premature beat resulted in retrograde conduction through the Kent bundly only. This was followed by antegrade A-V conduction through the His bundle, resulting in the first ventricular complex of the tachycardia. An example is given in figure 51. In patient H a tachycardia could not reproducibly be initiated by a single left ventricular premature beat.

Termination of tachycardias in WPW type A

By way of the synchronizing circuit of our stimulator premature beats were induced during the tachycardia following every eighth tachycardia complex. This was done till either the tachycardia was terminated or the atrial or ventricular tissue became refractory to the premature stimulus.

a. Atrial premature beats

Right atrial premature beats
In patients E and G the tachycardia, showing antegrade His conduction, could readily be terminated by a single early right atrial premature beat.

In patient D this could only be done by way of two right atrial premature beats given in close succession (fig. 52).

In patients F and H neither one nor two right atrial premature beats could terminate the tachycardia. This could only be done from the right atrium by driving at rates above the tachycardia frequency' ('overdriving').

In patient G the influence of premature beats on the tachycardias showing antegrade Kent conduction could not be studied. These tachycardias were too shortlived (8-17 beats) to permit accurate synchronization of the premature stimulus.

Left atrial premature beats
In three patients (F, G and H) where this was studied a single early left atrial premature beat promptly resulted in termination of the tachycardia (see fig. 53).

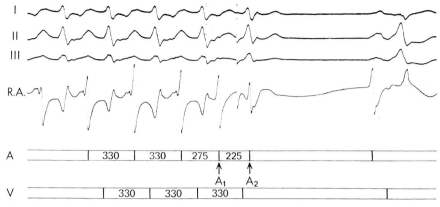

Fig. 52. Patient D. Termination of tachycardia by way of two right atrial premature beats (A₁ and A₂) given in close succession. The first atrial premature beat shortens the refractory period of the atrium, enabling the second one to reach and invade the tachy cardia circuit.

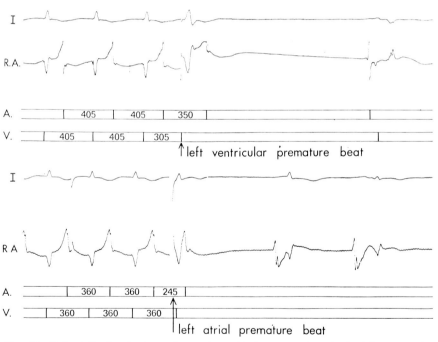

Fig. 53. Patient F. Termination of a tachycardia by way of a single left ventricular and left atrial premature beat (lower half of the figure). These observations were made during catheterizations on two different days. As shown in this figure the tachycardia frequency was not the same.

b. Ventricular premature beats

Right ventricular premature beats
In patients D, F and H the tachycardia could not be terminated by a single right ventricular premature beat.

In patient E the tachycardia could easily be terminated by a single right ventricular premature beat.

In patient G the tachycardias showing antegrade conduction by way of the His bundle could be terminated by a single right ventricular premature beat (see fig. 54).

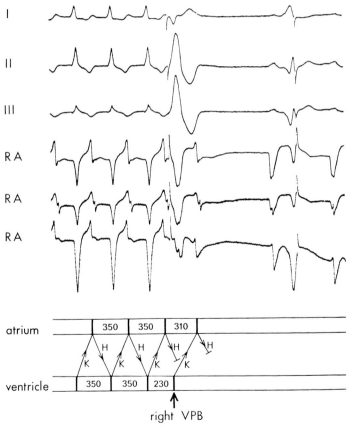

Fig. 54. Patient G. Termination of a tachycardia by way of a single right ventricular premature beat.

Influence of a single, right ventricular premature beat on the tachycardias showing antegrade conduction via the Kent bundle could not be studied, again, because these tachycardias were too shortlived to permit accurate synchronization of the premature stimulus.

Left ventricular premature beats
In three patients (F, G and H) where this was studied a single early left ventricular premature beat could always terminate the tachycardia. An example is given in figure 53 and figure 55.

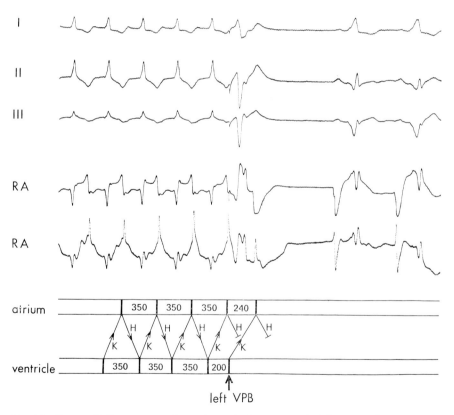

Fig. 55. Patient G. Termination of a tachycardia by one single left ventricular premature beat.

Influence of induced atrial and ventricular premature beats on the time relations of the tachycardia

a. Right atrial premature beats
The interval following the induced right atrial premature beat was fully compensatory in all patients studied.

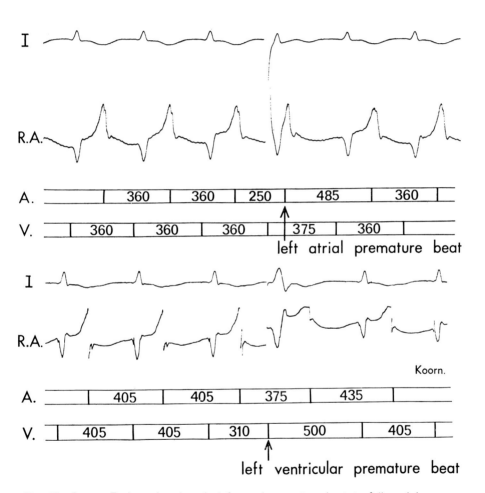

Fig. 56. Patient F. An induced early left atrial premature beat is followed by ventricular activation at a later time than expected during the tachycardia. The left ventricular premature beat does not influence the time relations of the tachycardia. As shown in fig. 53 shortening the premature beat interval with 5 msec results in termination of the tachycardia.

b. Left atrial premature beats

In patients F and G an early left atrial premature beat was followed by ventricular activation at a later time than expected during the tachycardia. An example is given in figure 56. For an explanation of this finding see under discussion. In both patients the tachycardia could be terminated by a single left atrial premature beat given after a shorter interval (see fig. 53).

Patient H: when during the tachycardia a premature beat was induced 90 to 75 msec after atrial activation, ventricular activation followed at an

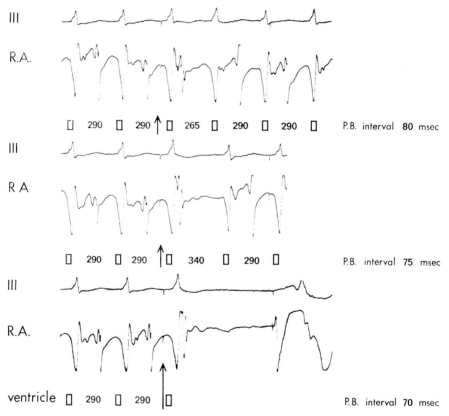

Fig. 57. Patient H. Lead III and an intracavitary lead from the right atrium are shown. **Top:** A left atrial premature beat given during the tachycardia after an interval of 80 msec is conducted to the ventricles, resulting in shortening of one R-R interval (265 msec). The next R-R interval has the usual cycle length of the tachycardia. **Middle:** A left atrial premature beat given after an interval of 75 msec is followed by a RR interval, longer than the cycle length of the tachycardia. **Bottom:** A left atrial premature beat given after an interval of 70 msec terminates the tachycardia.

earlier time than expected during the tachycardia (see fig. 57). A premature beat given after an interval of 75 msec, resulted in ventricular activation after an interval slightly longer than the tachycardia cycle (see fig. 57). Premature beats given after an interval of 70 msec resulted in termination of the tachycardia (fig. 57). The results in patient H suggest that at a premature beat interval from 90 to 75 msec a part of the tachycardia cycle can be preexcited, resulting in shortening of one tachycardia cycle. Apparently however, at an interval of 75 msec to 70 msec the atrial premature beat enters the A-V junction when this is still partly refractory from the foregoing impulse, resulting in slowing of transmission through the A-V junction (this becomes manifest by the interventricular interval following this premature beat, being longer than the cycle-length of the tachycardia).

c. Right ventricular premature beats
During the tachycardia the interval following the induced right ventricular premature beat was fully compensatory in all patients studied.

d. Left ventricular premature beats
In the three patients studied (F, G and H) a single left ventricular premature beat induced during the tachycardia was always followed by a fully compensatory interval.

Simultaneous registration of left and right atrial activation during the tachycardia

This was done in patients F and H, during a tachycardia showing antegrade conduction by way of the His bundle. Care was taken to position the recording electrodes close to the A-V ring. In both patients activation of the left atrium occurred much earlier than that of the right atrium. In patient F the beginning of left atrial activation preceded the beginning of right atrial activation by 80 msec, in patient H by approximately 100 msec (see fig. 58).

Discussion

The use of systematic electrical stimulation of the hearts of patients who have the Wolff-Parkinson-White syndrome and suffer from tachycardias have enabled us to study the mechanism of initiation and termination of supraventricular tachycardias in these patients. The results of our stimulation

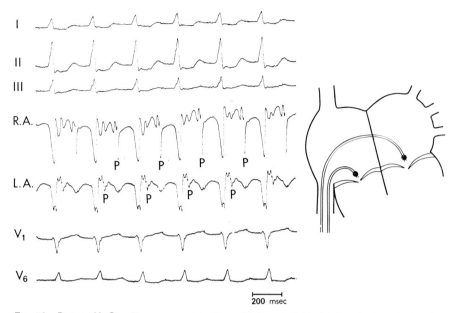

Fig. 58. Patient H. Simultaneous registration of left and right atrial activation during the tachycardia. Left atrial activation precedes the right atrial one by approximately 100 msec. Atrial activation is indicated by P.

studies done in patients with Wolff-Parkinson-White syndrome type A reveal that:

1. In W.P.W. type A it is easy to initiate and terminate a tachycardia by way of a single premature beat from the *left* side of the heart, while (in contrast with patients with W.P.W. type B) this could frequently not be accomplished from the *right* side of the heart.

2. In two patients simultaneous registration of left and right atrial intracavitary complexes from regions which are 'symmetrical' in respect to the atrial septum, during a tachycardia with antegrade A-V conduction by way of the His bundle showed that left atrial activation preceded right atrial activation by a considerable amount of time (80 and 100 msec.).

3. In those patients where regular driving was performed at the same rate from right and left atrium, the greatest amount of pre-excitation was seen during left atrial stimulation.

These results are in agreement with a circus movement or reciprocal mechanism by way of the A-V junction-His pathway and the anomalous A-V connection as a causal mechanism for tachycardias in W.P.W. type A.

Besides they speak in favour of a left sided location of the anomalous A-V connection in patients with Wolff-Parkinson-White syndrome type A. Our results indicate that Boineau and Moore's (5) finding that W.P.W. syndrome type A in the dog heart is the result of an accessory bundle connecting the right atrium and right ventricle at the posterior side of the heart, cannot be applied to the cases we studied.

As shown in our patient E apart from the previously reported initiating mechanisms (35) (atrial premature beat, ventricular premature beat and atrial echo beat) a tachycardia can be initiated by a ventricular echo beat.

In patient G an early atrial premature beat induced during right and left atrial driving, repeatedly resulted in a tachycardia with QRS complexes showing a maximal amount of pre-excitation. As shown in the intra-atrial leads, there was a 1 to 1 relation between atrial and ventricular activation. The frequency of this tachycardia was 200/min. Unfortunately the period of tachycardia lasted only 8 to 17 QRS complexes. This made it impossible to study the influence of atrial and ventricular premature beats on the tachycardia. Therefore, although it seems likely, definite proof that this tachycardia represents a circus movement tachycardia with antegrade A-V conduction by way of the Kent bundle and ventriculo-atrial conduction via the His bundle-A-V junction is lacking.

In patient G the induction of a ventricular premature beat during right or left ventricular driving repeatedly resulted in a tachycardia with antegrade A-V conduction by way of the A-V node-His bundle pathway. The way in which this type tachycardia could be initiated and terminated demonstrated that this was a true circus movement tachycardia.

In a patient with Wolff-Parkinson-White syndrome, type B we found (31) that during a tachycardia a properly timed atrial and ventricular beat could shorten one cycle length of the tachycardia. All following cycles were shifted to an earlier time than would be expected without shortening of one cycle by the premature beat.

According to Wenckebach and Winterberg (149) and Scherf et al. (126) no circus movement can be present when an induced premature beat is followed by a compensatory pause.

As described in chapter 2, if one wants to use this criterion in a fair way, however, one has to realize that even if one induces atrial and premature beats up to the refractory period of atrium and ventricle, it will not always be possible to reach the tachycardia circuit prior to the moment of passing by of the next tachycardia impulse. It depends on:

1. The distance between the site of stimulation and the tachycardia pathway.
2. The conduction properties of the tissue between the site of stimulation and the tachycardia pathway.
3. The frequency of the tachycardia and its resulting refractory period.
4. The spatial dimension of the tachycardia pathway.

Electrical stimulation from the right side of the heart and the left ventricle did not influence the time relations during the tachycardia in any of our patients.

A left atrial premature beat shortened one cycle of the tachycardia with a shift of the following tachycardia cycles to an earlier time in one of our patients (patient H).

Further shortening of the premature beat interval however resulted in an interventricular interval slightly longer than the tachycardia cycle. Termination of the tachycardia in this patient resulted at a premature beat interval of 70 msec.

Lengthening of the interventricular interval, following an early left atrial premature beat, making it longer than the tachycardia cycle, was also seen in patients F and G. This finding can be explained by assuming that the atrial premature beat enters the A-V junction, while this is still partly refractory from the foregoing impulse, resulting in marked slowing of transmission through the A-V junction. This explanation was given by Pick and Dominguez (111) for a similar finding in A-V junctional tachycardias. They noted in a patient with A-V junctional tachycardia and interference dissociation that an atrial complex during the tachycardia was sometimes followed by a ventricular complex, appearing after an interventricular interval longer than the tachycardia interval. They considered this ventricular complex the result of a 'captured' atrial beat. In view of the fact that contrary to the usual shortening of the interventricular interval following an atrical capture, now the interventricular interval measured longer than the tachycardia interval, they introduced for this finding the name 'delayed capture'. On further shortening of the premature beat interval the prematurely induced atrial impulse finds the A-V junctional tissue refractory, is therefore not transmitted through the A-V junction but makes the A-V junction refractory for the next impulse of the tachycardia. This results in termination of the tachycardia.

The finding that only left atrial premature beats influenced the time relations of the tachycardia are another argument that the anomalous A-V connection is situated on the left side of the heart. As pointed out above several factors influence the outcome of premature beats on the time relations of a circus movement tachycardia.

It remains to be demonstrated whether the fact that only left atrial premature beats could influence the time-relations of the tachycardias in our patients means that the spatial dimensions of the circus movement are rather small and that the anomalous A-V connection in patients with Wolff-Parkinson-White syndrome type A is situated not far from the A-V junction.

NORMAL PR INTERVAL - SMALL DELTA WAVE - NORMAL QRS COMPLEX

Variant forms of pre-excitation have been attributed to abnormal A-V connections originating from or located close to the A-V junction (Burch and Kimball (11), Lev et al. (75), Scherf and Cohen (127), Durrer et al. (35).

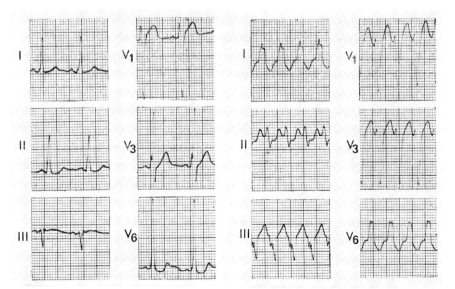

Fig. 59. Patient I. ECG during sinus rhythm (left) and tachycardia. See text.

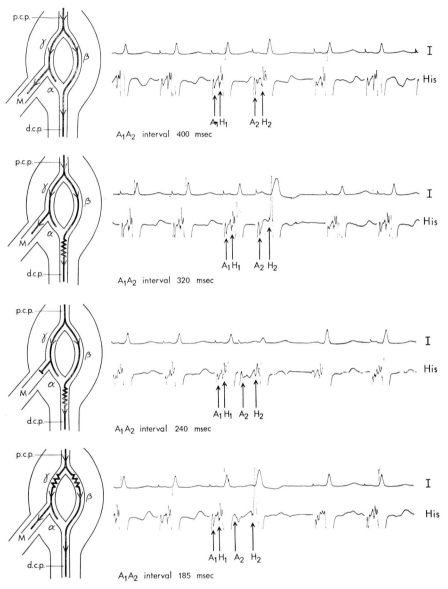

Fig. 60. Patient I. Changes in configuration of the QRS complex following a single right atrial premature beat (A₂) given during regular driving of the right atrium at progressively shorter premature beat intervals. As shown in the diagram on the left side of the figure we assume that the impulse after traversing a proximal common pathway (P.C.P.) reaches an area with two longitudinally dissociated pathways (β and γ). (Continued on p. 99)

We recently examined an 8 years old boy (patient I) who was referred to our department by Dr. M. Delstanche, Libramont, Belgium, for evaluation of attacks of palpitations since he was three years of age. Two or three times a year he suffered from an attack of rapid heart action lasting one to four hours. These attacks could not be prevented by digitalis or quinidine sulfate in a dosage of 75 mg three times daily. No abnormalities were found on physical examination. The chest X-ray showed a heart of normal size and configuration. The ECG between attacks showed (fig. 59) a regular sinus rhythm, frequency 100/min. The QRS axis was intermediate in the frontal plane. A small delta wave was present in lead I and V_3 to V_6. The interval between the beginning of the P wave and the beginning of the QRS complex measured 0.12 sec.

During the tachycardia the ECG showed (fig. 59) a ventricular frequency of 210/min. The QRS complex measured 0.12 sec. and had the configuration of a left bundle branch block. The QRS axis showed left axis deviation in the frontal plane. No definite P waves were seen. It was impossible from this ECG to decide between a supraventricular tachycardia with left aberrant conduction or a ventricular tachycardia caused by a focus in the right ventricle.

These pathways have different properties as far as refractoriness and conduction velocity are concerned. Pathway γ is connected with Mahaim fibres (M). The junction between the γ pathway and Mahaim fibre (M) is connected with a distal common pathway (D.C.P.) by pathway α. Pathway β is also connected with the distal common pathway. The latter pathway leads into the His bundle. Lead I and a His lead are shown at four selected premature beat intervals.

1. During regular driving with a BCL of 500 msec and at a premature beat interval of 400 msec the QRS complex is the result of fusion between conduction through pathway β and listal common pathway and conduction through γ pathway and Mahaim fibres. Conduction through pathway α arrives at the D.C.P. when this is already activated by way of pathway β.

2. At a premature beat interval of 320 msec slowing of impulse propagation in the distal common pathway results in an increased contribution to ventricular excitation by way of the Mahaim fibres. This is shown by the His bundle electrogram which merges into the first part of the QRS complex.

3. At a premature beat interval of 240 msec the impulse arrives so early at the site of origin of the Mahaim bundle that this area is still refractory. The impulse is conducted to the ventricles by the D.C.P. only.

4. At a premature beat interval of 185 msec slowing of the impulse proximal to the site of origin of the Mahaim bundle results in a QRS complex showing fusion between conduction through the anomalous pathway and the normal A-V conduction pathway. Ventricular excitation occurs for an important part by way of the Mahaim bundle as shown by the His bundle electrogram merging into the QRS complex.

Right atrial stimulation

During regular driving of the right atrium (BCL: 510 msec) every 8th stimulus was followed by a premature atrial beat. The premature beat interval was gradually shortened. Apart from lead I, II, III, V_1 and V_6, an intra-atrial lead (right atrium) and a His lead were registered. Gradual shortening of the right atrial premature beat interval resulted in changes in the configuration of the ventricular complex following this premature beat. This sequence is shown in figure 60 and 61. For the sake of clarity only lead I and the His lead are shown at characteristic premature beat intervals. Shortening of the premature beat interval resulted in a gradual increase in A-H interval (the interval between atrial activation and His bundle complex). As shown in figure 60 and 61, this was accompanied by a change in configuration of the QRS complex towards one as seen during the tachycardia. (Here only lead I and the His lead are shown. These changes towards a QRS configuration as seen during the tachycardia were present however in multiple simultaneous recorded leads).

The His bundle complex became buried into the beginning of the QRS complex at a premature beat interval of 320 msec. The QRS complex now looked similar to the QRS complexes during the tachycardia, indicating that during these attacks pre-excitation was present of at least a part of the ventricles by way of an anomalous conduction pathway.

On further shortening of the premature beat interval the amount of pre-excitation gradually diminished and His potentials preceding the QRS complex reappeared. At a premature beat interval of less than 250 msec pre-excitation disappeared.

At a premature beat interval of 210 msec. however, the QRS complexes showing an amount of pre-excitation became again discernible. Up to the refractory period of the right atrium (185 msec.) the induced premature beat was followed by a QRS complex, the A-H interval increasing to 230 msec. (it measured 50 msec. at the basic cycle length of 510 msec.).

It was repeatedly possible to induce a tachycardia at a premature beat interval of 200 to 210 msec. The way of initiation of the tachycardia had a characteristic pattern (see fig. 62). The atrial premature beat was followed by a QRS complex preceded by a His complex, partially buried into the QRS complex. This QRS complex showed some degree of pre-excitation. The QRS complexes of the tachycardia succeeding this induced premature beat were identical in configuration to the well known tachycardia of this patient (as shown in fig. 59).

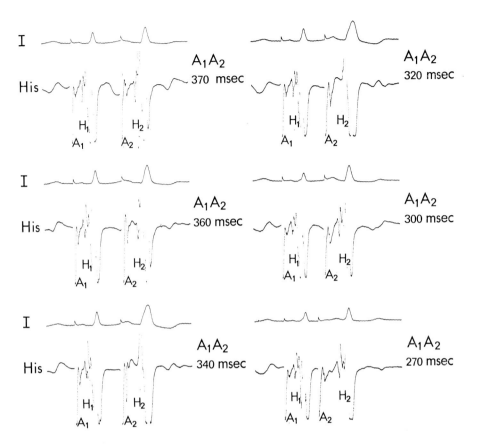

Fig. 61. Patient I. Selected examples of changes in configuration of the QRS on shortening the pramature beat interval from 370 msec to 270 msec. The recording of the His bundle electrogram is of help in determining the contribution to ventricular excitation by the Mahaim and His bundle. See also figure 60.

Both the configuration of the ventricular complexes following induced atrial beats and the way tachycardias could be initiated during atrial stimulation, can be explained by assuming:

1. The presence of Mahaim fibers running from the A-V node to the right side of the septum;
2. The presence of longitudinal dissociation in the A-V junction (fig. 60).

The gradual increase in contribution to ventricular excitation, by way of the

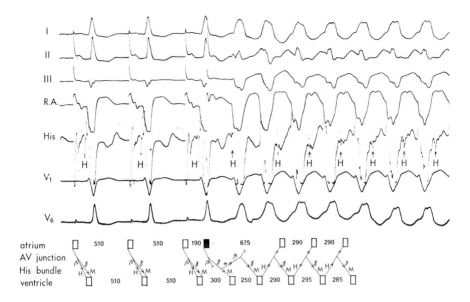

Fig. 62. Patient I. Initiation of a tachycardia by way of a single right atrial premature beat (premature beat interval 200 msec) during right atrial driving (BCL 510 msec). The possible mechanism is outlined in figure 63. Note that each ventricular complex during the tachycardia is followed by a His bundle electrocardiogram.

anomalous pathway on shortening the premature beat interval, can be explaned by a gradual lengthening in conduction time through the A-V node-His pathway distal to the take off of the Mahaim bundle (distal common pathway: d.c.p.) At a premature beat interval of 250 msec. however the impulse arrives at the Mahaim pathway when this is refractory. On further shortening the premature beat interval, retardation of impulse conduction takes place in the A-V junctional area, proximal to the site of origin of the Mahaim bundle. This results in arrival of the impulse at the Mahaim bundle at a time that this bundle is no longer refractory, resulting in a QRS complex showing fusion between conduction through the anomalous pathway and the normal A-V conduction pathway.

For this concept of retardation of impulse propagation at progressively higher levels of the specific conduction system on shortening the premature beat interval, no experimental data are as yet available, but it has been used for the explanation of other embarrassing findings like the unusual occurrence of incidental non-aberrantly conducted complexes in patients with atrial fibrillation and QRS complexes showing aberrant conduction (Wellens (146)) and for a 'gap' in A-V node transmission (Durrer et al. (33)).

At a premature beat interval of 200 to 210 msec. the QRS complex following the induced premature atrial beat has the aspect of a fusion complex between conduction through the anomalous pathway and the normal A-V conduction pathway. As can be seen in figure 62 the first QRS complex of the tachycardia is not preceded by a P wave nor by a His bundle electrogram. This is an important finding, showing that the first QRS complex of the tachycardia is not related to atrial activity but caused by re-entry into the proximal end of the anomalous bundle. A possible way to explain this re-entry phenomenon is shown in figure 63. It is based on the assumption that at a critical premature beat interval (200 to 210 msec.) impulse conduction is blocked in pathway β. This creates the possibility for the impulse after traversing slowly the γ and α pathway to re-enter the β pathway at its distal end. By way of the γ pathway the impulse reaches again the Mahaim bundle and activates the ventricle. As shown in the His lead (fig. 62) the first QRS complex of the tachycardia (250 msec after the QRS complex following the atrial premature beat) is followed by a His bundle electrogram. Thereafter the next QRS complex of the tachycardia follows. This suggests that after the initiation of the tachycardia the pathway during the tachycardia consists of either Mahaim bundle – His bundle – α pathway or Mahaim bundle – His bundle – β pathway – γ pathway (fig. 63).

Intracavitary leads from the right atrium showed that during the tachycardia a 1 to 1 relation was present between ventricular and atrial activation.

Right ventricular stimulation

During regular driving of the right ventricle with a basic cycle length of 400 msec. an induced ventricular premature beat given after an interval of 260 msec. reproducibly initiated a tachycardia (see fig. 64). This can be explained by assuming that at this premature beat interval the ventricular end of the Mahaim bundle is refractory. The impulse conducted by way of the His pathway only enters the reciprocal pathway in the A-V junction and is now able to pass through the A-V nodal end of the Mahaim bundle. The mechanism of the tachycardia thereafter being the same as described under right atrial stimulation.

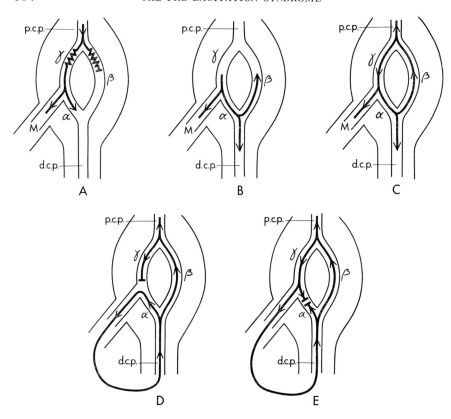

Fig. 63. Possible mechanism of initiation of tachycardia in patient I. Several stages of this mechanism are depicted. The premature atrial beat given after an interval of 200 msec finds pathway β refractory. It travels slowly through pathway γ, enters the Mahaim bundle and continues through pathway α to invade the D.C.P. (A). As shown in figure B this impulse may also enter the distal end of the β pathway and re-enter the γ pathway at its proximal end. After traversing the γ pathway the impulse activates the ventricle by way of the Mahaim bundle and continues its circulating course by entering the α pathway (C). We assume now that this α pathway is still refractory from the foregoing impulse. Ventricular excitation by way of the Mahaim bundle is followed by retrograde conduction into the His bundle. Thereafter two reciprocal pathways for maintaining a tachycardia are possible Either (fig. D) by way of the α pathway-Mahaim bundle and His bundle or (fig. E) by way of the β pathway-γ pathway-Mahaimbundle and His bundle.

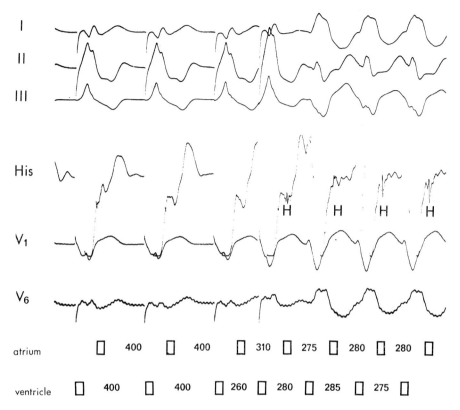

Fig. 64. Patient I. Initiation of a tachycardia by way of a single right ventricular premature beat during regular driving of the right ventricle. See text for discussion.

Influence of induced right atrial and right ventricular premature beats on the tachycardia

a. Right atrial premature beats

As indicated in figure 65 a single right atrial premature beat induced during the tachycardia resulted in a prematurely occurring QRS complex, identical to the complexes of the tachycardia. The interval following this complex was always less than fully compensatory.

Two induced right atrial premature beats given in close succession terminated the tachycardia (see fig. 66). Driving the right atrium at rates above the tachycardia frequency (driving frequency 240/min.) readily resulted in termination of the tachycardia.

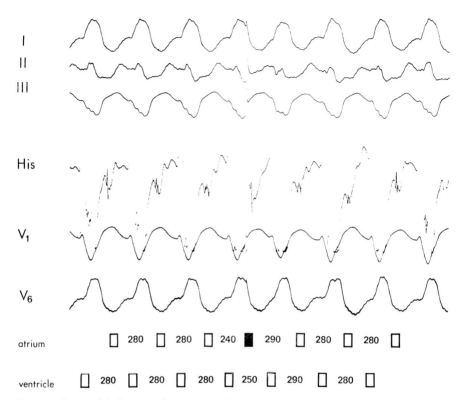

Fig. 65. Patient I. Influence of a single right atrial premature beat on the time relations of the tachycardia. Apparently the premature atrial beat pre-excites a part of the reciprocal pathway responsible for the tachycardia. The next tachycardia interval is less than fully compensatory.

b. Right ventricular premature beats

One electrically induced premature beat given during the tachycardia after an interval of 240 msec. or less, was followed by a tachycardia QRS complex at slightly less than a fully compensatory interval.

A single ventricular premature beat given after an interval of 210 msec. or less immediately terminated the tachycardia (see fig. 67).

Discussion

The way tachycardias could be initiated and terminated by atrial and ventricular premature beats, and the influence of induced atrial and ventricular

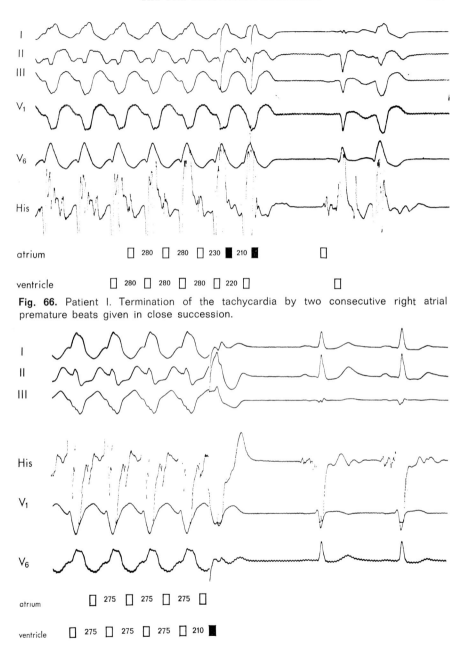

Fig. 66. Patient I. Termination of the tachycardia by two consecutive right atrial premature beats given in close succession.

Fig. 67. Patient I. Termination of the tachycardia by way of a single right ventricular premature beat.

premature beats on the time relations of the tachycardia, are in agreement with a circus movement as the causal mechanism for the tachycardias in this patient. The absence of atrial activity prior to the first beat of the tachycardia indicates that the atrium was not an essential part of the reciprocal pathway that initiated the tachycardia. The ECG during sinus rhythm and the changes in configuration of the QRS complex following the induction of right atrial premature beats suggest the existence in this patient of an abnormal connection between the A-V junction and the ventricle.

The recording of the His bundle electrogram enabled us to exclude the possibility that our patient suffered from A-V junctional tachycardias with left bundle branch block.

Abnormal connections between a part of the A-V junction and the ventricle have been described anatomically by Mahaim and Winston (85).

Figure 68 shows two possible pathways for circus movement tachycardias in patients with such an abnormal connection. In our patient tachycardias with normal QRS width were never recorded, nor could we initiate such a tachycardia during our stimulation studies. The ease by which tachycardias could be initiated during right ventricular driving suggests that unidirectional block in the Mahaim bundle might have been responsible for the absence of tachycardias showing a circus movement in the reversed direction.

As demonstrated in the previous pages, the mechanism of initiation of the

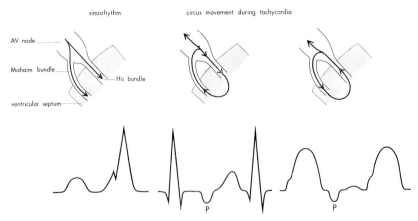

Fig. 68. Schematic representation of the possible pathway for circus movement tachycardias and their resulting electrocardiograms in patients with a Mahaim bundle between the A-V node and the ventricular septum.

tachycardia in our patient was a complex one. In order to account both for the configuration of the QRS complexes following atrial premature beats of different premature beats intervals and for the initiation of tachycardias following a single right atrial premature we had to take recourse in the explanation given above.

Although using accepted concepts like longitudinal dissociation in the A-V junction it is clear that our explanation is a conjectural one.

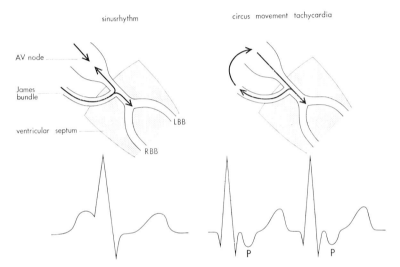

Fig. 69. Possible pathway of circus movement tachycardia in a patient with a James bundle.

SHORT PR - NORMAL QRS - SYNDROME

In 1968 Durrer (32) described a 38-year old woman with a very short PR interval (0.07 sec.) and normal QRS width (0.10 sec.). When right atrial stimulation was performed at the junction with the superior caval vein, the atrial complex was followed after 70 msec by the QRS complex. This proved that in this patient the short PR interval was not caused by a pacemaker located near the coronary sinus or in the atrioventricular node (a location already very unlikely because of the configuration of the P wave), but that sinus beats were conducted without appreciably delay to the ventricle.

Ventriculo-atrial conduction during right ventricular driving was very short as well (70-90 msec).

This case (our patient J) was the first functional demonstration of a bypass, short-circuiting at least a major part of the atrio-ventricular junction. The normal configuration and duration of the QRS complex suggested a close connection between the bypass tract and the tail of the A-V junction. Such muscular connections, entering the tail of the A-V junction, have been described anatomically by James (57). A schematic representation of the anatomic situation and the resulting electrocardiogram is given in figure 42 and 43. In figure 69 the possible pathway of a circus movement in such a situation is depicted.

As reported by Durrer (32), the patient suffered from supraventricular tachycardias with a 1 to 1 relation between atrial and ventricular complexes. The frequency of this tachycardia was 250/min (fig. 70). Such a tachycardia began during manipulation with the electrode catheter in the right atrium The onset of the tachycardia was followed by rapid deterioration of the condition of the patient. She perspired heavily and complained about substernal

RP interval 80 msec   RR interval 240 msec

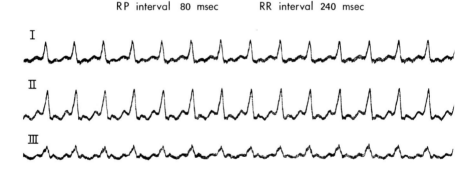

intracavitary lead middle R.A.

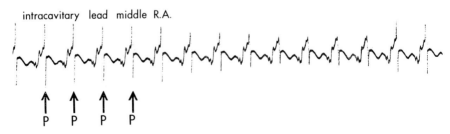

Fig. 70. Patient J. Supraventricular tachycardia, frequency 250/min. with 1 to 1 relation between atrial and ventricular rhythm. As described in the text it is not possible to differentiate between a circus movement tachycardia, an atrial tachycardia or an atrial flutter with 1 to 1 A-V conduction.

pain. No bloodpressure was obtainable. The tachycardia was therefore immediately converted to sinus rhythm by a single defibrillating shock of 100 Watt/sec.

In view of the dramatic change in her condition with the onset of the tachycardia, it was decided to terminate the catheterization, and not to study systematically the way tachycardias could be initiated and terminated.

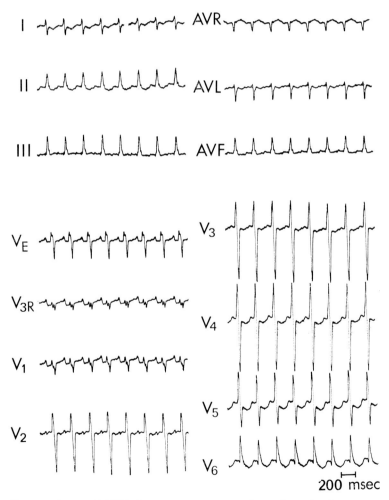

Fig. 71. Patient K. ECG showing a supraventricular tachycardia, frequency 220/min.

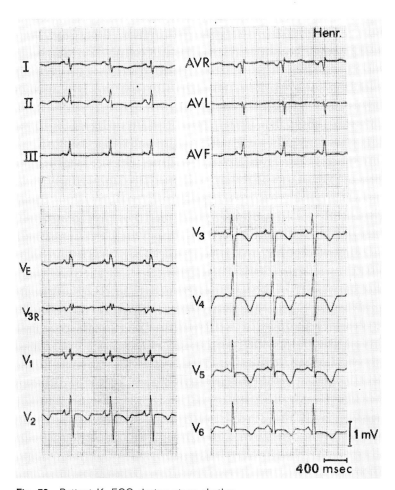

Fig. 72. Patient K. ECG during sinus rhythm.

It is possible that the tachycardia represents a true circus movement tachycardia by way of the A-V node, James bundle and a piece of atrial tissue (as shown in fig. 69). We cannot exclude however, that the tachycardia represented an atrial tachycardia or atrial flutter with 1 to 1 conduction to the ventricle.

We have recently studied another patient (K) with a short PR interval (0.12 sec.) and normal QRS complex. This 35-year old woman suffered from attacks of palpitations since she was 17 years old. The frequency and length of these attacks had gradually increased. The last year prior to admission she had one attack every two months lasting from one day to one week. She came to our department with an attack of tachycardia of 6 days' duration. It was unsuccessfully tried to terminate the tachycardia by quinidine 300 mg 6 times daily.

The electrocardiogram showed a supraventricular tachycardia; frequency 220/min (fig. 71). No definite P waves could be identified.
The ECG, after the tachycardia was terminated (fig. 72), showed a sinus rhythm, with a frequency of 80/min. The PR interval measured 0.12 sec. The depth of the terminal negative deflection of the P wave over the right precordium suggested left atrial enlargement. The QRS complex measured 0.09 sec and showed a rsr configuration over the right precordium. The PJ time measured 0.21 sec. The QT time was prolonged (0.4 sec). The T wave was negative in all leads except AVR. This finding was attributed to the combination of quinidine medication and a post-tachycardia syndrome. Immediately after admission, while she was having a tachycardia, the patient was studied.

The findings during the catheterization were:

1. Simultaneous intracavitary registration of left and right activation during the tachycardia revealed that left atrial activation preceded the right atrial one by approximally 80 msec (fig. 73).
2. The tachycardia could not be terminated by a single electrically induced premature beat given high or low in the right atrium, the left atrium or the right ventricle.
3. The induced premature beats were always followed by a fully compensatory interval.

The tachycardia ended when an early left atrial premature beat was followed by three, irregularly spaced, atrial complexes. The initiation of the tachycardia was studied by inducing premature beats during regular driving of the right and left atrium. A single premature beat, given high or low in the right atrium during regular driving of the right atrium up to the refractory period of the atrium, did not result in a tachycardia. The catheter was therefore advanced into the left atrium (it was possible to reach the left atrium through an open foramen ovale). Regular driving in the left atrium resulted in QRS complexes that differed from those following right atrial stimulation (see fig. 74).

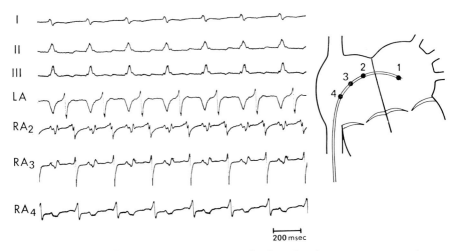

Fig. 73. Patient K. Simultaneous registration of left and right atrial activation during the tachycardia. Left atrial activation precedes the right atrial one by approximately 80 msec.

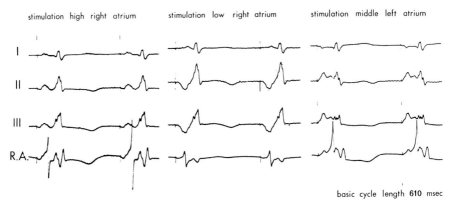

Fig. 74. Patient K. Differences in QRS configuration during regular driving of the right atrium at identical frequencies.

A single left atrial premature beat, given after an interval of 315 msec, was followed by a tachycardia (fig. 75). It is impossible to decide from the configuration of the QRS complex following the induced premature atrial beat, how during this complex, conduction to and through the ventricle

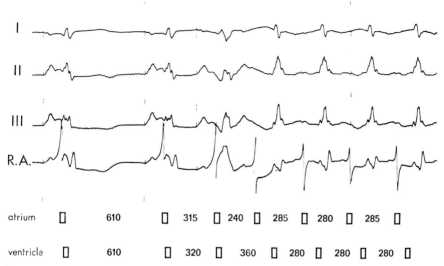

atrium	[]	610	[]	315	[]	240	[]	285	[]	280	[]	285	[]
ventricle	[]	610	[]	320	[]	360	[]	280	[]	280	[]	280	[]

Fig. 75. Patient K. Initiation of tachycardia by way of a single left atrial premature beat during regular driving of the left atrium. See text for discussion.

occurred. As shown in the intracavitary lead, this QRS complex is followed by an atrial complex.

Thereafter a tachycardia supervenes. Three explanations are possible as far as origin and mechanism of the tachycardia are concerned:

1. Left atrial tachycardia: The interval between the left atrial premature beat and the next atrial complex suggests the possibility of a left atrial tachycardia based upon a re-entry pathway located in the left atrium.

2. An A-V junctional tachycardia: One has to assume then that the atrial complex preceding the tachycardia following the induced left atrial premature beat, represents an A-V junctional echo beat and is followed by a reciprocal A-V junctional tachycardia. The fact that during the tachycardia left atrial activation precedes right atrial activation by 80 msec suggests that during the tachycardia retrograde conduction towards the atrium took place by way of the anomalous A-V connection. One therefore has to locate the impulse formation during the tachycardia in the A-V junction very close to the anomalous pathway.

3. A circus movement tachycardia: The presence of an abnormal A-V

connection opens the possibility of antegrade conduction through the A-V junction – His pathway and retrograde conduction through the anomalous connection. The initiating mechanism would be an atrial echo following the induced left atrial premature beat. (See also page 77). This atrial echo would find the anomalous A-V connection refractory and can only be conducted towards the ventricle by way of the A-V node – His pathway. This impulse, by entering the ventricular end of the anomalous A-V connection, could be retrogradely conducted towards the left atrium. By re-entering the atrial end of the A-V junction, the first cycle of the ensuing tachycardia would be completed.

As said before, it was impossible to terminate the tachycardia by a single premature beat from the right or left atrium or the right ventricle. Nor could we influence the time relations of the tachycardia by a single premature beat induced at any of these locations.

Considering these findings, one has to assume that if this were a reciprocal or circus movement tachycardia, the spatial dimensions of the tachycardia pathway are very small.

Our conclusion is that from the available data it is impossible to identify the mechanism responsible for the tachycardia in this patient.

After the tachycardia was initiated again and we failed to terminate it by a single premature beat given in the right or left atrium or in the right

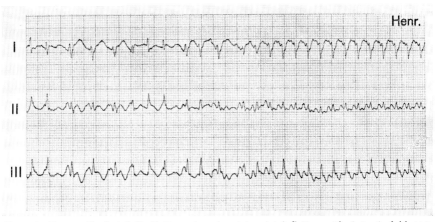

Fig. 76. Patient K. Atrial fibrillation changing into atrial flutter with 1 to 1 A-V conduction. Paper speed 25 mm/sec.

ventricle, it was decided to drive the right atrium at rates above the tachy-cardia frequency ('overdriving').

Shortly after driving the atrium at 300/min atrial fibrillation occurred. As shown in figure 76 this changed into atrial flutter with 1 to 1 conduction towards the ventricle. The RR interval measured 220 msec, indicating a ventricular rate of 270/min. The patient rapidly lost consciousness and had a grand mal seizure. She was immediately converted to sinus rhythm by a defibrillation shock of 100 Watt/sec.

Discussion

Incidence of and theories as to the origin of the syndrome of the short PR interval with normal configuration of the P wave and QRS complex are excellently reviewed by Scherf and Cohen (127). Among the many diseases in which this phenomenon has been described are coronary artery disease, with or without myocardial infarction, hypertension, beri-beri-heart disease, hyperthyroidism, acute rheumatic heart disease, psychiatric disorders and glycogen storage disease.

Both Clerc, Levy and Cristesco (17) and Lown, Ganong and Levine (83) described an increased incidence of paroxysmal tachycardias in patients with short PR intervals and normal P waves and QRS complexes.

Much discussion has centered around the question: Does a normal con-figuration of the P wave necessarily mean an origin in the sinus node or high in the right atrium? Scherf and Cohen (127) think that this is true, Katz and Pick (61) however do believe in a coronary nodal rhythm consisting of a normally configurated P wave with short PR interval and normal QRS complex. They assume that this rhythm originates near the mouth of the coronary sinus close to the tail of the sino-atrial node.

In the dog heart Moore et al. (104) demonstrated that activation of the atrium near the coronary sinus resulted in normal polarity of the P waves unless there was concomitant damage to the atrial myocardium.

These observations however, are not relevant to our two patients. Stimu-lation high in the right atrium, close to be the sinus node, resulted in very short PR intervals. The most attractive hypothesis to explain the short PR interval, is to assume the presence of a bypass short-circuiting the whole or an important part of the A-V junction. Such a connection, called the posterior internodal tract, has been described by James (57).

In patient K the QRS complexes following stimulation of the left atrium differed in configuration as compared to those resulting from right atrial stimulation. One could explain this finding by assuming as postulated by Sherf and James (133) that the direction of input from the atrium into the A-V conduction system determines the spread of excitation though the ventricular specific conduction system.

The validity of this concept however needs to be proven functionally by comparing the configuration of the QRS complexes following right and left atrial stimulation at identical rates at different stimulation sites in patients who do not show signs of pre-excitation.

Electrocardiograms appearing in articles reporting the outcome of right atrial stimulation at different stimulation sites (Leon et al. (74) and left atrial stimulation (Massumi and Tawakkol (91), Harris et al. (48), and Lau et al. (73)) failed to show such differences in QRS complex configuration.

This has also been our experience in six patients where the presence of an atrial septal defect enabled us to perform right and left atrial stimulation at identical driving rates.

From clinical electrocardiograms we know that changes in QRS configuration following markedly different P waves are extremely unusual (Somlyo and Grayzel (136), Scherf and Cohen (127), Mirowski (97), Frankl and Soloff 39)).

We think that in our patient K the most likely possibility is that the anomalous A-V connection is running from the left atrium to an area very close to the tail of the A-V junction. The QRS complexes following atrial stimulation are fusion complexes resulting from conduction through the A-V junctional pathway and the anomalous A-V connection.

Normally the properties of the A-V junction serve to protect the ventricle against too rapid atrial rhythms. As demonstrated in our patients the presence of an A-V bypass leading to the functional absence of the whole or a major part of the A-V junction creates a life-threatening situation when rapid atrial rhythms (like atrial flutter or atrial fibrillation) supervene.

It is not surprising that two patients from Lown's series (83) died suddenly. Both of these were subject to paroxysms of atrial fibrillation.

CONCLUSIONS

In this chapter we reported our observations on initiation and termination of tachycardias in patients with the pre-excitation syndrome.

Based upon the outcome of electrical stimulation from different sites of the heart we have postulated in our patients the most likely location of their anomalous A-V connection and the mechanism responsible for their tachycardias.

Recently new therapeutic possibilities (electrical stimulation of the heart or surgical interruption of the tachycardia pathway) have been advanced for the treatment of those patients whose tachycardias cannot be controlled by drug therapy.

Both ways of therapy are still in an investigational state. In order to facilitate in the future the correct decision as to the therapy to be chosen, we feel that at present the following work-up in these patients is necessary.

(1) Based upon the routine electrocardiogram and using Lev-Ferrer's scheme of possible anomalous A-V connections (fig. 42 and 43) all theoretical ways that can lead to the particular electrocardiogram of the patient should be considered. In the evaluation of the electrocardiogram the interval between the beginning of the P-wave and the delta-wave, and the width of the QRS complex deserve special attention. It is important to realize that identical electrocardiograms can be the result of different types of anomalous A-V connections.

This has been demonstrated by Lev et al. (75). They found that an electrocardiographic pattern compatible with W.P.W. syndrome type B was caused by an A-V nodal bypass tract (James bundle) and paraspecific fibers (Mahaim fibers) running on the right side of the intraventricular septum.

If in a patient a short PR interval and a delta-wave are followed by a QRS complex of less than 0.12 sec in duration a septal, ventricular insertion of the anomalous A-V connection seems very probable.

(2) If two different A-V pathways are functionally present ventricular excitation starts at two different points. When the properties of these pathways as far as refractoriness and conduction velocity are concerned, are not identical, increasing the heart rate or induction of premature atrial beats will augment these differences. This will lead to changes in the contribution in ventricular excitation from each of the two pathways, resulting in definite changes in the QRS complex.

As we have demonstrated in the previous pages stimulation of the atrium close to the anomalous A-V connection increases the amount of pre-excitation. This knwledge can be of help in locating the atrial end of the anomalous A-V connection.

When an increase in heart rate by electrical stimulation of the atrium or an electrically induced premature atrial beat does not result in any or only minimal changes in the QRS complex, ventricular excitation by way of the anomalous A-V connection only, or a long common proximal pathway of A-V conduction (like in Mahaim fibers) becomes very likely.

The induction of atrial premature beats with gradually decreasing interval will also identify the group of patients with the pre-excitation syndrome where the refractory period of the anomalous A-V connection is so short that the ventricle is a helpless victim if rapid atrial rhythms like atrial flutter or atrial fibrillation occur. We feel that patients with these properties of their A-V bypass live under the constant threat of sudden death.

(3) Initiation and termination of the tachycardias should be studied carefully, preferably with help of electrical stimulation. This is of value in the localization of the abnormal A-V connection and a necessity if one considers to use electrical stimulation to terminate and prevent tachycardias on a long-term basis. The value of registering the influence of electrically induced atrial and ventricular premature beats on the length of one ventricular cycle during the tachycardia remains to be proven. It seems logical at this time that a cycle of a circus movement of large spatial dimensions can easily be invaded and shortened by an appropriately timed atrial or ventricular premature beat. If this is true, this phenomenon could be helpful in differentiating between tachycardias using an anomalous A-V connection located far away from the A-V junction and tachycardias where an A-V bypass tract situated close to the A-V node is part of the reciprocal pathway.

(4) Both during pre-excitation and tachycardias endocardial leads should be used in an effort to localize grossly the earliest point of ventricular excitation during pre-excitation and atrial excitation during the tachycardia. Observations on the revived perfused human heart (Durrer et al. (34)) and stimulation studies by Massumi et al. (92) suggest that ventriculo-atrial conduction by way of the A-V node results in almost simultaneous excitation of the right and left atrium. Excitation of the left atrium well in advance of the right atrium during the tachycardia suggests a location of the atrial end of the anomalous A-V connection on the left side of the heart.

We want to stress that exact localization of the abnormal A-V connections by way of endocardial leads alone, is extremely difficult if not impossible. Even with biplane X ray equipment the exact site of the catheter point in relation to the endocardial surface can not be determined accurately.

After these four points have been studied it is usually possible to come to a gross localization of the anomalous A-V connection and to conclude on the mechanism responsible for the tachycardia. If the tachycardias cannot be treated satisfactorily by drug therapy we would favour at present the following therapeutic approach.

If the outcome of the stimulation studies suggests a location of the anomalous A-V connection in or close to the A-V junction, electrical therapy seems to be treatment of choice (if it can be demonstrated that it is possible to terminate the tachycardia by way of electrically induced premature beats).

An anomalous A-V connection situated relatively far away from the A-V junction should preferably be treated by surgical interruption of the abnormal A-V pathway. It is essential that prior to this procedure both the ventricular and the atrial end of the anomalous connection should be localized. This should be done by a careful search for the earliest point of excitation on the ventricle and on the atrium during electrical stimulation of respectively the atrium and the ventricle. In the W.P.W. type A due to the localization of the anomalous A-V connection on the posterior side this can be a very difficult procedure. In these patients Dreifus et al. (28) and Edmunds et al. (37) interrupted the tachycardia pathway by dissecting the A-V node. This operation should also be used in patients with abnormal A-V connections, located close to the A-V node, where tachycardias can not be controlled by electrical stimulation of the heart. In view of the fact that conduction through the anomalous A-V connection is frequently intermittent in character, this procedure has to be accompanied by implantation of a pacemaker.

One should realize however, that if the anomalous A-V connection lies lateral to the area where the A-V node dissection is made, very rapid ventricular rates following very rapid atrial rhythms are still possible. This point stresses again the necessity to be informed about the properties of the anomalous A-V connection prior to the operation.

CHAPTER 7

ELECTRICAL STIMULATION OF THE HEART IN THE TREATMENT OF TACHYCARDIAS

It is possible to distinguish at present five different modes of electrical stimulation for the treatment of patients whose tachycardias cannot satisfactory be controlled by drug therapy.

1. The delivery of an appropriately timed single or two consecutive premature beats at the site (atrium or ventricle) where this results in termination of the tachycardia.
2. Paired depolarisation of the heart by the use of paired stimulation or coupled pacing.
3. Simultaneous stimulation of the atrium and ventricle.
4. Regular driving of the heart at rates above the frequency of the tachycardia: 'Overdriving'.
5. Regular driving of the heart for the prevention of paroxysmal supraventricular and ventricular tachycardias.

The method to be chosen will depend upon the type and mechanism of the tachycardia that has to be treated.

1. The delivery of an appropriately timed single or two consecutive premature beats at the site (atrium or ventricle) where this results in termination of the tachycardia

This method can be used in patients with reciprocal tachycardias. Its effectiveness is ascribed to the creation of refractoriness in a part of the reciprocal pathway responsible for the tachycardia. The feasibility of this method has been demonstrated in supraventricular tachycardia (Barold et al. (3)), A-V junctional tachycardia (Coumel et al. (22, 23), Hunt et al. (55), Goldreyer and Bigger (42) and tachycardias related to the pre-excitation syndrome (Durrer et al. (31), Massumi et al. (30), Cobb et al. (18), and Ryan et al. (120)).

New examples of the termination of A-V junctional tachycardias by a single or two consecutive premature beats are given in chapter 5. The importance of careful determination of the site where (atrium or ventricle, left or right) and the interval after which a premature stimulus should be given is clearly demonstrated by our experience in patients with the Wolff-Parkinson-White syndrome (chapter 6). All the observations mentioned above were made during short term catheterization studies. The practical problem, however, is how to use this principle on a long term basis?

The most ideal apparatus for this purpose would be an implantable pacemaker, able to give an electrical stimulus during the tachycardia after a pre-set interval (as determined during the work-up prior to the insertion of the pacemaker). For safety it should only be possible to give such a stimulus once after every 6th or 8th ventricular complex. External application of a magnet over the pacemaker generator could be used to switch the pacemaker on when needed. It is obvious that we do not have such 'demand' pacemakers at present. Ryan and coworkers (120) however, invented an ingenious way to apply a similar principle in their patient with W.P.W. type A.

They positioned an electrode catheter in the right ventricle and connected the electrode with a demand pacemaker. This pacemaker (American Optical Company) could be converted from demand to fixed rate pacing by holding a magnet near the generator pocket. This fixed rate stimulation producing competitive pacing was continued till one of the pacemaker stimuli fell at the correct interval after a tachycardia complex, thereby terminating the tachycardia.

2. *Paired depolarisation of the heart by the use of paired stimulation or coupled pacing*

Introduced in 1963 by Lopez et al. (82), paired stimulation is done by driving the heart at a regular rate with two closely spaced stimuli. The second stimulus is thereby timed to occur so early in the relative refractory period of the first complex, that it results in electrical depolarisation without mechanical contraction.

This can also be obtained by coupled pacing. Depending upon the level where one wants to apply this technique, an early stimulus is given after every atrial or ventricular complex. This stimulus is applied at such a time interval that the same result is reached as described above for the second stimulus during paired stimulation.

These techniques have been used for the treatment of supraventricular and ventricular tachycardias (Chardack et al. (15), Braunwald et al. (6, 7), Langendorf and Pick (69), Meijler and Durrer (95), Scheppokat et al. (123), Büchner (10)).

The possible hazard of precipitating ventricular fibrillation while attempting to place the second stimulus after the appropriate interval has limited the clinical usefullness of this type stimulation at the ventricular level.

3. *Simultaneous stimulation of the atrium and ventricle*

If a circus movement with consecutive activation of atria and ventricles is responsible for the tachycardia, simultaneous activation of both atrium and ventricle will prevent the occurrence of such tachycardias. This was proven by Coumel et al. (23), in two patients suffering from reciprocal A-V junctional tachycardias. They connected the negative pole of their pacemaker with an electrode attached epicardially to the right ventricle. The positive pole was connected with an electrode sewn to the right atrium. The thereby accomplished simultaneous driving of the right atrium and ventricle at a rate of 100/min resulted in complete prevention of tachycardias.

It is clear that a similar method can be successfully applied to patients with the pre-excitation syndrome and circus movement tachycardias. It seems particularly useful in those patients where the termination of a reciprocal tachycardia is immediately followed by a new bout of tachycardia (like in our patient G from chapter 5).

4. *Regular driving of the heart at rates above the frequency of the tachycardia: 'Overdriving'*

As shown by Haft et al. (44), Lister et al. (81), and Zeft et al. (157), it is possible to terminate tachycardias by driving the heart at rates above the tachycardia frequency. This method can and is successfully applied in patients with atrial tachycardias, atrial flutter, A-V junctional tachycardias and tachycardias in patients with the pre-excitation syndrome.

The possible mechanisms responsible for this effect are:

a. suppression of an ectopic focus by driving at rates above the discharge rate of the ectopic focus.

b. the creation of refractoriness in a part of the pathway of reciprocal tachycardias.

c. induction of a short period of unstable atrial fibrillation followed by conversion to sinus rhythm. (this phenomenon is frequently seen during 'overdriving' of atrial flutter).

Rapid atrial pacing for the treatment of supraventricular tachycardias has three advantages over electrocardioversion:

a. there is no need for anaesthesia.

b. no antiarrhythmic agents are necessary.

c. it can be used without hazard in patients with digitalis overdosage.

If it is not possible to terminate the tachycardia by driving the heart at rates above the tachycardia frequency, the deliberate induction of atrial fibrillation by this method can be benificial. The induction of atrial fibrillation is accompanied by concealed conduction in the A-V junction resulting in a drop in ventricular rate. The presence of atrial fibrillation also eases the use of digitalis for further reduction in transmission of atrial impulses through the A-V junction. An example of an intractable atrial tachycardia benefiting from the electrical induction of atrial fibrillation, is given by Wiener and Dwyer (150).

At present it is impossible to use demand 'overdrive' therapy on a long term basis, since no such pacemakers are commercially available. We want to warn against the deliberate use of the 'overdrive' principle as long as one has not excluded the possibility of a pre-excitation syndrome in the patient presenting with a tachycardia. Rapid stimulation of the atrium frequently results in atrial flutter or atrial fibrillation. As pointed out before (chapter 6) this can be a very hazardous and immediately life-threatening if the refractory period of the anomalous A-V connection is very short.

At this point it is important to stress that before one decides to drive the heart at very high rates, one should carefully identify the exact location of the tip of the stimulating electrode.

A defibrillator should always be immediately available.

5. *Regular driving of the heart for the prevention of paroxysmal supraventricular and ventricular tachycardias*

We know that slow heart rates (resulting from sino-auricular block, sinus bradycardia, slow A-V junctional rhythm and total heart block) favour the development of atrial and ventricular tachyarrhythmias. Han et al. (47) showed that the incidence of ectopic rhythms is directly related to the basic rate of the heart. They (46) also found that asynchrony of recovery of excitability of atrial and ventricular muscle increases on slowing the heart rate, favouring the development of arrhythmias due to focal re-excitation (see also chapter 2).

This knowledge has led to the use of cardiac pacing in the treatment of tachyarrhythmias both at the supra-ventricular and ventricular level. The purpose of this therapy is to reduce the asynchrony of recovery of excitability and to shorten the time interval during which muscular tissue is able to respond to a stimulus from an ectopic center.

At the supraventricular level the frequent occurrence of tachycardias (mostly atrial flutter or atrial fibrillation) in patients with sinus bradycardia, S-A block and slow A-V junctional rhythm, has led to the introduction of the term brady-tachycardia-syndrome. Examples of the benificial effect of cardiac pacing in these patients both from the atrium and ventricle have been given by Cohen et al. (20), Cheng (16), Hornbaker et al. (54), Slama et al. (135) and Zipes et al. (158).

At the ventricular level acute and chronic recurrent tachyarrhythmias can occur in the presence of normal A-V conduction. When these arrhythmias cannot satisfactorily be controlled by drug therapy or when optimal drug therapy results in bradycardia with or without impairment of A-V conduction, cardiac pacing can be life saving.

Electrical driving of the heart has been used under these circumstances both on a short and long term basis. The cause of the ventricular tachyarrhythmias varied from acute myocardial infarction, chronic coronary artery disease, cardiac surgery and electrolyte imbalance to intoxication by digitalis and other drugs.

Cardiac pacing was accomplished in these patients both endo- and epicardially from the right and left atrium and the right ventricle (Sowton et al. (137, 138), Heiman and Helwig (51), Mc Callister et al. (93), Cohen et al. (21), Schoonmaker et al. (130), Beller et al. (4) Kastor et al. (59), Woodson et al. (155), De Francis and Giordano (27), Morris et al. (49), Moss et al. (105), Lew and March (77), and Zipes et al. (158), Burchell and Merideth (14)). It was frequently necessary, even with optimal drug therapy, to drive the heart at rates above 100/min. to suppress ectopic activity. If this had to be done on a long term basis a fixed rate pacemaker had to be inserted.

In those patients where optimal pharmacologic therapy suppressed ectopic activity, but resulted in slow ventricular rates, a demand pacemaker could be used.

As already mentioned if one intends to implant a definite pacemaker to prevent recurrent tachyarrhythmias in a patient, the site of stimulation should be chosen carefully. At first sight the most ideal location for pacing in patients with normal A-V conduction who suffer from ventricular tachyarrhythmias seems to be at the atrial level. When however a re-entry mechanism is responsible for the arrhythmia the direction of spread of excitation through the ventricle might play a role in the creation of the re-entry pathway. This is demonstrated by the finding in one of our patients that a ventricular tachyarrhythmia could not be controlled by driving the right atrium at a rate of 110/min (with a 1 to 1 A-V conduction) but completely suppressed by driving the right ventricule at a frequency of 85/min.

One should also realize (as pointed out by Sowton et al. (138) that the concommitant administration of anti-arrhythmic drugs in these patients might impair A-V conduction. Prior to implanting the definite pacemaker one should therefore always study, with help of a temporary pacing unit, the ideal pacing site (atrium or ventricle) and the effect of the combined use of atrial pacing and drug administration on A-V conduction. This also enables one to chose the correct pacing rate that prevents arrhythmias at rest and during moderate exercise. In those patients where disturbances in A-V conduction become manifest during this period, a ventricular pacemaker should be implanted.

Conclusion

At present five different methods of electrical stimulation of the heart are available for the treatment of tachycardias that do not respond to pharmacologic therapy.

We want to stress that a careful investigation into the type and mechanism of the tachycardia is essential before making a decision on the method to be used.

SUMMARY

In order to treat a patient with a tachycardia correctly and to give a well founded opinion upon the most likely etiology and prognosis, identification of the site of origin of the tachycardia (atrium, A-V junction or ventricle) is mandatory. This requires a knowledge of the electrocardiographic characteristics of different types of tachycardia, based upon rhythm, frequency, relation between atrial and ventricular activation and QRS complex configuration and width. In addition the value of the typical signs on physical examination that accompany a certain type of tachycardia and the response to carotid sinus massage should be known. In this way the origin of the majority of tachycardias can be diagnosed. Unfortunately it is impossible to make a diagnosis, however, in those patients who present with a regular tachycardia, with an electrocardiogram, showing wide QRS complexes without definite P waves and who do not respond to carotid sinus massage. In this group of patients the only possible way to make a diagnosis is to utilise additional diagnostic procedures.

1. Intra-esophageal and intra-atrial leads to identify atrial activity and its relation to ventricular activity.
2. The recording of potentials from the specific conduction system.
3. The use of electrical stimulation of the heart.

Apart from their site of origin, tachycardias can be classified according to their mechanism. Traditionally they have been divided into those resulting from a rapidly discharging focus and those caused by a reciprocal or re-entry mechanism.

As discussed in chapter 2 our knowledge of the electrophysiological mechanisms leading to the initiation and maintenance of focal tachycardias is small. More is known about the mechanisms causing a reciprocal or re-entry tachycardia. Essential is the presence of two functionally dissociated pathways which are connected with each other at their proximal and distal end. A critically timed impulse can find one of the pathways refractory at its proximal end, travel through the other pathway and via the distal communication return into the first pathway. This sequence can lead to an echo beat followed by a reciprocal or re-entry tachycardia. The tachycardia will end when the circulating impulse in its pathway collides with refractory tissue. Such a situation can frequently be created by eliciting an appropriately timed premature beat during the tachycardia. In order to make a diagnosis of a reciprocal tachycardia one should therefore be able to demonstrate that such a tachycardia can be initiated and terminated by a single premature beat.

Theoretically it was thought possible to differentiate between focal and reciprocal tachycardias by recording the effect of premature beats on the time relations of the tachycardia. While it was accepted that a complex of a tachycardia occurring after a shorter than expected interval would be in favour of a reciprocal tachycardia, it was postulated that no reciprocal or circus movement mechanism could be present, when a premature beat did not influence the time relations of the tachycardia. We want to stress that this theory is only valid, however, if one is able to induce a premature beat early enough to reach the focus or reciprocal pathway prior to the moment of discharge, or passage of the next impulse of the tachycardia. As shown in chapter 2 it is frequently not possible to fulfill this criterion. The spatial dimension of a reciprocal pathway may differ considerably or it may be situated in a protected area such as the A-V junction. This can make it impossible to stimulate close enough to the reciprocal pathway to demonstrate that this, and not a focus, was actually responsible for the tachycardia. With the technique of stimulation we used it is therefore not possible to exclude a very small reciprocal pathway if the results favour the presence of an ectopic focus. Our material consisted of six patients with atrial flutter, seven with A-V junctional tachycardia and eleven with tachycardia in the presence of a pre-excitation syndrome.

The purpose of our study was to estimate the value of electrical stimulation of the heart in the elucidation of the origin and mechanisms of these tachycardias and for treatment. All patients were studied in the catheterization room using two or more electrode catheters.

Stimulation was performed with a safe and reliable stimulator, enabling us to give three independent stimuli (one driving stimulus, creating a regular basic rhythm and two testing stimuli eliciting premature beats) either separately or in combination. The interval after which the testing pulse was applied could either be started by the driving stimulus or by feeding the electrical activity of the heart itself into a synchronizer. The duration of the stimuli was kept at 2 msec. Current strength was less than twice the diastolic threshold current.

The results of our stimulation studies in patients with atrial flutter suggested that either an unprotected focus or a reciprocal rhythm situated in a very small area low in the atrium was responsible for the dysrhythmia. We could find no evidence supporting the theory that atrial flutter is the result of a circus movement involving a large part of the atrium. We did not find it possible to terminate the atrial flutter with a single atrial premature beat or two atrial premature beats given in the closest possible succession. This was in marked contrast to our results in patients with A-V junctional tachycardia.

In all seven patients with A-V junctional tachycardia one or two premature beats terminated the tachycardia. As stated before for the differentiation of a focal or at a reciprocal origin of the tachycardia the study of the initiation of the tachycardia was found to be mandatory. In the four patients where this was done, the results favoured a reciprocal mechanism.

The results in our 8 patients with 'classical' Wolff-Parkinson-White syndrome (W.P.W.) supported the theory of a circus movement mechanism. In five patients with the W.P.W. syndrome type A we found that a tachycardia could easily be initiated and terminated by a single premature beat from the left side of the heart.

In contrast with patients with W.P.W. type B, this could frequently not be accomplished from the right side of the heart.

In two patients with W.P.W. type A, during a tachycardia showing antegrade A-V conduction by way of the His bundle, left and right atrial intracavitary complexes were registered simultaneously from regions which were 'symmetrical' with respect to the atrial septum. This showed that left atrial activation preceded right atrial activation by a considerable length of time. In those patients with W.P.W. type A where regular stimulation was applied at the same rate from the right and the left atrium, the greatest degree of pre-excitation was seen during left atrial stimulation. Our results are in favour of a left sided location of the anomalous A-V connection in patients with Wolff-Parkinson-White syndrome type A.

In one patient with W.P.W. type A we found that a tachycardia could be initiated by way of a ventricular echo beat. In another patient with W.P.W. type A an early premature beat induced during right and left atrial stimulation repeatedly resulted in a tachycardia with QRS complexes showing a maximal amount of pre-excitation. It is very likely that this represents a circus movement tachycardia with antegrade A-V conduction by way of the Kent bundle and ventriculo-atrial conduction via the His bundle A-V junction. When atrial and ventricular premature beats were applied during the tachycardia in patients with W.P.W. type A, only left atrial premature beats were found to influence the time relations of the tachycardia. It remains to be demonstrated whether this finding means that the spatial dimensions of the circus movement during the tachycardia are rather small and that the anomalous A-V connection in patients with W.P.W. syndrome type A is situated not far from the A-V junction.

One patient was studied in whom the results favoured a Mahaim bundle between the A-V node and the right side of the interventricular septum. The changes in configuration of the QRS complexes following the induction of right atrial premature beats during right atrial stimulation and the mechanism of initiation of a tachycardia in this patient could only be explained by assuming a complex anatomical and electrophysiological architecture of the A-V junction.

Two patients with a short PR interval and a normal QRS complex were studied. This pattern was thought to be the result of an A-V bypass entering close to the A-V node at its junction with the bundle of His. Both patients demonstrated the dangers inherent in the functional absence of the whole or a major part of the A-V junction when rapid atrial rhythms supervened. Using electrical stimulation from different sites of the heart it was possible to postulate the most likely location of the anomalous A-V connection and the mechanism responsible for the tachycardia in patients with the pre-excitation syndrome. We think that these investigations are essential for making a decision about treatment, (surgery versus electrical stimulation) in patients with the pre-excitation syndrome whose tachycardia cannot be satisfactorily controlled by drug therapy.

Five different methods of electrical stimulation are presently available for the treatment of tachycardias:

1. The delivery of an appropriately timed single or two consecutive premature stimuli at the site (atrium or ventricle) where this will result in termination of the tachycardia.
2. Paired depolarisation of the heart using paired stimulation or coupled pacing.
3. Simultaneous stimulation of the atrium and ventricle.

4. Regular stimulation of the heart at rates above the frequency of the tachycardia: 'overdriving'.
5. Regular stimulation of the heart to prevent paroxysmal supraventricular and ventricular tachycardias.

The method which is choosen will depend upon the site of origin and the mechanism of the tachycardia. If electrical therapy on a long term basis is to be considered the site, pattern and rate of stimulation should be first carefully determined with a temporary pacing unit. Our study demonstrates that electrical stimulation of the heart can be very helpfull, both in the elucidation of the origin and of some of the mechanisms responsible for the tachycardia and for its treatment.

REFERENCES

1. ALANIS, J., GONZALEZ, H. and LOPEZ, E. (1958). Electrical activity of the bundle of His. *J. Physiol.* 142:127.
2. ALEXANDER, S. and PING, W.C. (1966). Fatal ventricular fibrillation during carotid sinus stimulation. *Amer. J. Cardiol.* 18:289.
3. BAROLD, S. S., LINHART, F. W., SAMET, P. and LISTER, F. W. (1969). Supraventricular tachycardia initiated and terminated by a single electrical stimulus. *Amer. J. Cardiol.* 24:37.
4. BELLER, B. M., FRATER, R. W. M. and WULFSOHN, N. (1968). Cardiac pacemaking in the management of post operative arrhythmias. *Ann Thorac. Surg.* 6:68.
5. BOINEAU, J. P. and MOORE, E. N. (1970). Evidence for propagation of activation across accessory atrioventricular connection in types A and B pre-excitation. *Circulation* 41:375.
6. BRAUNWALD, E. ROSS, J., JR., and SONNENBLICK, E. H. (1964). Clinical observations on paired electrical stimulation of the heart, *Amer. J. Med.* 37:700.
7. BRAUNWALD, N. S., GAY, W. A., JR., MORROW, A. G., and BRAUNWALD, E. (1964). Sustained paired electrical stimuli: Slowing of the ventricular rate and augmentation of contractile force. *Amer. J. Cardiol.* 14:385.
8. BROWN, B. and ACHESON, G. (1952). Aconitine induced auricular arrhythmias and their relation to circusmovement flutter. *Circulation* 6:529.
9. BROWN, W. H. (1936). A study of the oesophageal lead in clinical electrocardiography. *Amer. Heart J.* 12:1.
10. BUCHNER, M. (1969). Zur Physiologie und Pathophysiologie der Erregungsbildung im menschlichen Herzen. *Arch. Kreislaufforschg.* 60:327.
11. BURCH, G. E. and KIMBALL, F. L. (1946). Notes on the similarity of QRS complex configuration in the W.P.W. syndrome. *Amer. Heart J.* 32:560.
12. BURCHELL, H. B. and STURM, R. E. (1967). Electroshock hazards. *Circulation* 35:227.
13. BURCHELL, H. B., FRYE, R. L., ANDERSON, M. W., and McGOON, D. C. (1967). Atrioventricular and ventriculo-atrial excitation in W. P. W. syndrome (type B) Temporary ablation at surgery. *Circulation* 36:663.
14. BURCHELL, H. B., and MERIDETH, J. (1969). Management of cardiac tachyarrhythmias with cardiac pacemakers. *Ann. N.Y. Ac. Sci.* 167:546.
15. CHARDACK, W. M., GAGE, A. A., and DEAN, D. C. (1965). Paired and coupled stimulation of the heart. *Bull. N.Y. Acad. Med.* 41:462
16. CHENG, T. O. (1968). Transvenous ventricular pacing in the treatment of paroxysmal atrial tachyarrhythmias alternating with sinus bradycardia and standstill. *Amer. J. Cardiol.* 22:874.
17. CLERC, A., LEVY, R., and CRISTESCO, C. (1938). A propos du raccourcissement permanent de l'espace P-R de l'electrocardiogramme sans deformation du complexe ventriculaire. *Arch. Mal. Coeur* 31:569.

18. COBB, F. R., BLUMENSCHEIN, S. D., SEALLY, W. C., BOINEAU, J. P., WAGNER, G. S. and WALLACE, A. G. (1968). Succesfull surgical interruption of the bundle of Kent in a patient with Wolff-Parkinson-White syndrome.

19. COELHO, E., DA FONSECA, J. M. and NUMES, A. (1950). Les altérations du potential intra-auriculaire. *Cardiologia* 17:346.

20. COHEN, H. E., KAHN, M., and DONOSO, E. (1967). Treatment of supraventricular tachycardias with catheter and permanent pacemaker. *Amer. J. Cardiol.* 20:735.

21. COHEN, L. S., BUCCINO, R. A., MORROW, A. G. and BRAUNWALD, E. (1967). Recurrent ventricular tachycardia and fibrillation treated with a combination of beta adrenergie blockade and electrical pacing. *Ann. Inter. Med.* 66:945.

22. COUMEL, PH., CABROL, C., FABIATO, A., GOURGON, R., and SLAMA, R. (1967). Tachycardia permanente par rythme réciproque. *Arch. Mal. Coeur* 60:1830.

23. COUMEL, PH., MOTTE, G., GOURGON, R., FABATIO, A., SLAMA, R., and BOUVRAIN, Y. (1970). Les tachycardies supraventriculaires par rythme réciproque en dehors du syndrome de Wolff-Parkinson-White. *Arch. Mal, Coeur* 63:35.

24. VAN DAM, R. TH., DURRER, D., STRACKEE, J., and VAN DER TWEEL, L. H. (1956). The excitability of the dog's left ventricle, determined by anodal, cathodal and bipolar stimulation. *Circulation Res.* 4:196.

25. VAN DAM, R. TH. (1960). *Experimenteel onderzoek naar het prikkelbaarheidsverloop van de hartspier.* Amsterdam, thesis.

26. DAMATO, A. N., LAU, S. H., STEIN, E., BERKOWITZ, W. D., and COHEN, S. J. (1969). Study of atrio-ventricular conduction in man using electrode catheter recordings of His bundle activity. *Circulation* 39:287.

27. DE FRANCIS, N. A., and GIORDANO, R. A. (1968). Permanent epicardial atrial pacing in the treatment of refractory ventricular tachycardia. *Amer. J. Cardiol.* 22:742.

28. DREIFUS, L. S., NICHOLS, H., MORSE, O., WATANABE, Y. and TRUEX, R. (1968). Control of recurrent tachycardia of W. P. W. syndrome by surgical ligature of the A-V bundle. *Circulation* 38:1030.

29. DRESSLER, W. (1966). Prolonged depressing effect of premature supraventricular beats. *Amer. Heart J.* 72:25.

30. DURRER, D. and ROOS, J. P. (1967). Epicardial excitation of the ventricles in a patient with W.P.W. syndrome. *Circulation* 35:15.

31. DURRER, D., SCHOO, L., SCHUILENBURG, R. M. and WELLENS, H. J. (1967). The role of premature beats in the initiation and the terminiation of supraventricular tachycardias in the W.P.W. syndrome. *Circulation* 36:644.

32. DURRER, D. (1969). Electrical aspects of human cardiac activity: a clinical, physiological approach to excitation and stimulation. *Cardiovasc. Res.* 2:1.

33. DURRER, D., SCHUILENBURG, R. M., and WELLENS, H. J. J. (1969). The role of the A-V junction in the genesis of arrhythmias in the human heart. *Proc. Kon. Acad. Wet. Series C.* 72:501.

34. DURRER, D., VAN DAM, R. T., FREUD, G. E., JANSE, M. J., AERZBACHER, R. and MEIJLER, F. L. (1970). Total excitation of the isolated heart. *Circulation* 41:899.

35. DURRER, D., SCHUILENBURG, R. M., and WELLENS, H. J. J. (1970). Pre-excitation revisited. *Amer. J. Cardiol.* 25:690.

36. EASLY, R. M., JR., and GOLDSTEIN, S. (1968). Differentiation of ventricular tachycardia from junctional tachycardia with aberrant conduction: The use of competitive atrial pacing. *Circulation* 37:1015.

37. EDMONDS, J. H., ELLISON, G. G., and CREWS, T. L. (1969). Surgically induced atrioventricular block as treatment for recurrent atrial tachycardia in W.P.W. syndrome. *Circulation* 39: suppl. I :105.

38. FERRER, M. J. (1967). New concepts relating to the pre-excitation syndrome. *J. Amer. med. Ass.* 201:162.
39. FRANKL, W. S., and SOLOFF, L. A. (1968). Left atrial rhythm: Analysis by intra-atrial electrocardiogram and the vector cardiogram. *Amer. J. Cardiol.* 22:645.
40. GETTES, L. S. and YOSHONIS, K. F. (1970). Rapidly recurring supraventricular tachycardia: A manifestation of reciprocating tachycardia and an indication for propanolol therapy. *Circulation* 41:689.
41. GIRAUD, G., PUECH, P., LATOUR, H., and HERTAULT, J. (1960). Variations de potentiel lieés a l'activité du systeme de conduction auriculo-ventriculaire chez l'homme. *Arch. Mal. Coeur.* 53:575.
42. GOLDREYER, B. N. and BIGGER, J. TH. (1969). Spontaneous and induced re-entrant tachycardia. *Ann. intern. Med.* 70:87.
43. GREENWOOD, R. J., and DUPLER, D. A. (1962). Death following carotid sinus pressure. *J. Amer. med. Ass.* 181:605.
44. HAFT, J. I., KOSOWSKY, B. D., LAU, S. H., STEIN, E. and DAMATO, A. N. (1967). Termination of atrial flutter by rapid electrical pacing of the atrium. *Amer. J. Cardiol.* 20:239.
45. HAN, J., and MOE, G. K. (1964). Non-uniform recovery of excitability in ventricular muscle. *Circ. Res.* 14:44.
46. HAN, J., MILLET, D., CHIZZONITTE, B., and MOE, G. K. (1966). Temporal dispersion of recovery of excitability in atrium and ventricle as a function of heart rate. *Amer. Heart. J.* 71:481.
47. HAN, J., DE TRAGLIA, J., MILLET, D., and MOE, G. K. (1966). Incidence of ectopic beats as a function of basic rate in the ventricle. *Amer. Heart J.* 72:632.
48. HARRIS, B. C., SHAVER, J. A., GRAY, S., KROETZ, F. W., and LEONARD, J. J. (1968). Left atrial rhythm. Experimental production in man. *Circulation* 37:1000.
49. HARRIS, P. D., MALM, J. R., BOWMAN, F. O., HOFFMANN, B. F., KAISER, G. A., and SINGLER, D. H. (1968). Epicardial pacing to control arrhythmias following cardiac surgery. *Circulation* 37: suppl. 11 :178.
50. HECHT, H. H. (1946). Potential variations of the auricular and right ventricular cavities in man. *Amer. Heart J.* 32:39.
51. HEIMAN, D. F., and HELWIG, J., JR. (1966). Suppression of ventricular arrhythmias by transvenous intracardiac pacing. *J. Amer. med. Ass.* 195:1150.
52. HOFFMAN, B. F., and CRANEFIELD, P. F. (1964). The physiological basis of cardiac arrhythmias. *Amer. J. Med.* 37:670.
53. HOFFMAN, B. F. (1966). The genesis of cardiac arrhythmias. *Progr. cardiovasc. Dis.* 8:319.
54. HORNBAKER, J. H. J., O'NEAL HUMPHRIES, J., and ROSS, R. S. (1969). Permanent pacing in the absence of heart block: an approach to the management of intractable arrhythmias. *Circulation* 39:189.
55. HUNT, N. C., COBB, F. R., WAXMAN, M. B., ZEFT, H. J., PELER, R. H., and MORRIS, J. J. (1968). Conversion of supraventricular tachycardias with atrial stimulation: evidence for re-entry mechanism. *Circulation* 38:1060.
56. JAMES, T. N. (1961). Morphology of the human atrio ventricular node with remarks pertinent to its electrophysiology. *Amer. Heart. J.* 62:756.
57. JAMES, T. N. (1963). The connecting pathways between the sinus node and A-V node and between the right and left atrium. *Amer. Heart J.* 66:498.
58. JANSE, M. J., VAN DER STEEN, A. B. M., VAN DAM, R. TH., and DURRER, D. (1969). Refractory period of the dog's ventricular myocardium following sudden changes in frequency. *Circulation Res.* 24:251.
59. KASTOR, J. A., DE SANCTIS, R. W., HARTHORNE, J. W., and SCHWARTZ, G. H. (1967).

Transvenous atrial pacing in the treatment of refractory ventricular irritability. *Ann. intern. Med.* 66:939.

60. KATZ, L. N., and PICK, A. (1956). *Clinical electrocardiography Part I. The arrhythmias.* Philadelphia, Lea and Febiger.

61. KATZ, L. and PICK, A. (1960). Current status of theories of mechanism of atrial tachycardia, flutter and fibrillation. *Prog. cardiovasc. Dis.* 2:650.

62. KISHON, Y., and SMITH, R. E. (1969). Studies in human atrial flutter with the use of proximity electrodes. *Circulation* 40:513.

63. KISTIN, A. D. (1961). Retrograde conduction to the atria in ventricular tachycardia. *Circulation* 24:236.

64. KISTIN, A. D. (1966). Problems in the differentiation of ventricular arrhythmia from supraventricular arrhythmia with abnormal QRS. *Progr. cardiovasc. Dis.* 9:1.

65. KISTIN, A. D., TAWAKKOL, A., and MASSUMI, R. A. (1967). Atrial rhythm in ventricular tachycardia, occuring during cardiac catheterization. *Circulation* 35:10.

66. KOSSMAN, CH., RADER, B., BERGEN, A., BRUMLIK, J., and BRILLER, S. A. (1950). Electrograms in atrial flutter, atrial tachycardia and atrial fibrillation. *First World Congr. Cardiol., Paris.*

67. LANARI, A., LAMBERTIN, A., and RAVIN, A. (1956). Mechanism of experimental atrial flutter. *Circ. Res.* 4:282.

68. LANGE, G. (1965). Action of driving stimuli from intrinsic and extrinsic sources on in situ cardiac pacemaker tissue. *Circ. Res.* 17:449.

69. LANGENDORF, R., and PICK, A. (1965). Observations on the clinical use of paired electrical stimulation of the heart. *Bull. N.Y. Acad. Med.* 41:535.

70. LATOUR, H., and PUECH, P. (1957. *Electrocardiographie endocavitaire.* Paris, Masson.

71. LATOUR, H., PUECH, P., and HERTAULT, J. (1962). L'echo (conduction réciproque) en cours de tachycardie ventriculaire. *Arch. Mal. Coeur.* 55:180.

72. LAU, S. H., DAMATO, A. N., BERKOWITZ, W. D., and PATTON, R. D. (1969). A study of atrioventricular conduction in atrial fibrillation and flutter in man using His bundle recordings. *Circulation* 40:71.

73. LAU, S. H., COHEN, S. J., STEIN, E., HAFT, J. J., ROSEN, K. M., and DAMATO, A. N. (1970). P waves and P loops in coronary sinus and left atrial rhythms. *Amer. Heart J.* 79:201.

74. LEON, D. F., LANCASTER, J. E., SHAVER, J. A., KROETZ, F. W., and LEONARD, J. J. (1970). Right atrial ectopic rhythms. Experimental production in man. *Amer. J. Cardiol.* 25:6.

75. LEV, M., LEFFLER, W. B., LANGENDORF, R., and PICK, A. (1966). Anatomic findings in a case of ventricular pre-excitation (W.P.W.) terminating in complete atrioventricular block. *Circulation* 34:718.

76. LEV, M. (1966). Anatomic considerations of anomalous A-V pathways. In: Dreifus, L.S. and Likoff, W. (eds) *Mechanisms and therapy of cardiac arrhythmias.* New York, Grune and Stratton. p :665.

77. LEW, H. T., and MARCH, H. W. (1967). Control of recurrent ventricular fibrillation by transvenous pacing in the absence of heart block. *Amer. Heart J.* 73:794.

78. LEWIS, T., FEIL, M., and STROUD, W. (1920). Observations upon flutter and fibrillation. II The nature of auricular flutter. *Heart* 7:191.

79. LEWIS, T., DRURY, A. N., and ILIESCU, C. C. (1921). A demonstration of circus movement in clinical flutter of the auricles. *Heart* 8:341.

80. LINHART, J. W., BRAUNWALD, E., and ROSS, J., JR. (1965). Determinants of the

refractory period of the atrioventricular nodal system in man. *J. clin. Invest.* 44:883.

81. LISTER, J. W., COHEN, L. S., BERNSTEIN, W. H., and SAMET, P. (1968). Treatment of supraventricular tachycardias by rapid atrial stimulation. *Circulation* 38:1044.

82. LOPEZ, J. F., EDELIST, A., and KATZ, L. N. (1963). Slowing of the heart rate by artifical electrical stimulation with pulses of long duration in the dog. *Circulation* 28:759.

83. LOWN, B., GANONG, W. F., and LEVINE, S. A. (1952). The syndrome of short PR interval, normal QRS complex and paroxysmal rapid heart activation. *Circulation* 5:539.

84. LOWN, B., KLEIGER, R., and WILLIAMS, J. W. (1965). Cardioversion and digitalis drugs. Changed threshold to electric shock in digitalis animals. *Circ. Res.* 17:519.

85. MAHAIM, J., and WINSTON, M. R. (1941). Recherches d'anatomie comparée et de pathologie experimentale sur les connections hautes de faisceau de His et Tawara. *Cardiologia* 5:189.

86. MALINOW, M. R., and LANGENDORF, R. (1948). Different mechanisms of fusion beats. *Amer. Heart J.* 35:448.

87. MARQUES, M., MOTA, J., and NOQUEIRA, R. (1962). The mechanism of atrial flutter. *Cardiologia* 40:269.

88. MARRIOT, H. J. L., and ROGERS, H. M. (1969). Mimics of ventricular tachycardia, associated with the W.P.W. syndrome. *J. Electrocardiol.* 2:77.

89. MASSUMI, R. A., TAWAKKOL, A. A., KISTIN, A. D. (1967). Revaluation of electrocardiographic and bedside criteria for diagnosis of ventricular tachycardia. *Circulation* 36:628.

90. MASSUMI, R. A., KISTIN, A. D., and TAWAKKOL, A. A. (1967). Termination of reciprocating tachycardia by atrial stimulation. *Circulation* 36:637.

91. MASSUMI, R., and TAWAKKOL, A. A. (1967). Direct study of left atrial P waves. *Amer. J. Cardiol.* 20:331.

92. MASSUMI, R. A., SARIN, R. K., TAWAKKOL, A. A., RIOS, J. C., and JACKSON, H. (1969). Time sequence of right and left atrial depolarization as a guide to the origin of the P waves. *Amer. J. Cardiol.* 24:28.

93. MC. CALLISTER, B. D., MC. GOON, D. C., and CONNOLLY, D. C., (1966). Paroxysmal ventricular tachycardia and fibrillation without complete heart block. Report of a case with an permanent internal cardiac pacemaker. *Amer. J. Cardiol.* 18:848.

94. MEREDITH, J., and TITUS, J. C. (1968). The anatomic connections between sinus and A-V node. *Circulation* 37:566.

95. MEIJLER, F. L., and DURRER, D. (1965). Physiological and clinical aspects of paired stimulation. *Bull. N.Y. Acad. Med.* 41:575.

96. MINES, G. R. (1913). On dynamic equilibrium in the heart. *J. Physiol.* 46:23.

97. MIROWSKI, M. (1966). Left atrial rhythm. Diagnostic criteria and differentiation from nodal arrhythmias. *Amer. J. Cardiol.* 17:203.

98. MIROWSKI, M., and ALKAN, W. J. (1967). Left atrial impulse formation in atrial flutter. *Brit. Heart. J.* 29:299.

99. MIROWSKI, M. (1967). Ectopic rhythm originating anteriorly in the left atrium. Analysis of twelve cases with P wave inversion in all precordial leads. *Amer. Heart J.* 74:299.

100. MOE, G. K., PRESTON, J. B., and BURLINGTON, H. (1956). Physiologic evidence for a dual AV transmission system. *Circ. Res.* 4:357.

101. MOE, G. K., ABILDSKOV, J. A., and HAN, J. (1964). Factors responsible for the initiation and maintenance of ventricular fibrillation. In *Sudden Cardiac Death* :p 56. Edit by Surawicz, B. and Pellegrino, E. D. New York, Grune and Stratton.

102. MOE, G. K., MENDEZ, C., and HAN, J. (1965). Aberrant A-V impulse propagation in the dog heart: A study of functional bundle branch block. *Circulation Res.* 16:261.
103. MOE, G. K. and MENDEZ, C. (1966). The physiologic basis of reciprocal rhythm. *Progr. cardiovasc. Dis.* 8:461.
104. MOORE, E. N., JOMAIN, S. L., STUCKEY, J. H., BUCHANAN, J. W., and HOFFMAN, B. F. (1967). Studies on ectopic atrial rhytrms in dogs. *Amer. J. Cardiol.* 19:676.
105. MOSS, A., RIVERS, R. J., GRIFFITH, L. S. C., CARMEL, J. A., and MILLARD, E. B. Jr. (1968). Transvenous left atrial pacing for recurrent ventricular fibrillation. *New Engl. J. Med.* 278:928.
106. NARULA, O. S., SCHERLAG, B. J., and SAMET, P. (1970). Pervenous pacing of the specialized conduction system in man: His bundle and A-V nodal stimulation. *Circulation* 41:77.
107. OEHNELL, R. F. (1944). Pre-excitation, a cardiac abnormality. *Acta med. Scand. Suppl.* 152.
108. PAES, DE CARVALHO, A., and ALMEIDA, D. F. (1960). Spread of activity through the atrioventricular node. *Circ. Res.* 8:801.
109. PICK, A., LANGENDORF, R., and KATZ, L. N. (1951). Depression of cardiac pacemakers by premature impulses. *Amer. Heart J.* 41:49.
110. PICK, A., and KATZ, L.N. (1955). Disturbances of impulse formation and conduction in the pre-excitation (W.P.W.) syndrome. Their bearing on its mechanism. *Amer. J. Med.* 19:759.
111. PICK, A., and DOMINGUEZ, P. (1957). Non paroxysmal A-V nodal tachycardia. *Circulation* 16:1022.
112. PICK, A., and LANGENDORF, R. (1960). Differentiation of supraventricular and ventricular tachycardias. *Progr. Cardiovasc. Dis.* 2:391.
113. PICK, A., LANGENDORF, R., and KATZ, L. N. (1961). A-V nodal tachycardia with block. *Circulation* 24:12.
114. PICKERS, B. A., GOLDBERG, M. J. and WATSON, C. C. (1969). Termination of a tachyarrhythmia by paired pacing. *Brit. Med. J.* 2:161.
115. PORUS, R. L., and MARCUS, F. J. (1963).Ventricular fibrillation during carotid-sinus stimulation. *New. Engl. J. Med.* 268:1338.
116. PRINZMETAL, M., CORDAY, E., BRILL, J. C., OBLATH, R. W., and KRUGER, H. E. (1952). *The auricular arrhythmias.* Springfield, Charles C. Thomas.
117. ROSEN, K. M., LAU, S. H., and DAMATO, A. N. (1969). Simulation of atrial flutter by rapid coronary sinus pacing. *Amer. Heart J.* 78:635.
118. ROSENBAUM, F. F., HECHT, H. H., WILSON, F. N., and JOHNSTON, F. D. (1945). Potential variations of the thorax and the esophagus in anomalous atrio ventricular excitation. (W.P.W.). *Amer. Heart J.* 29:281.
119. ROSENBLUETH, A., and GARCIA RAMOS, J. (1947). Studies on flutter and fibrillation. II The influence of artificial obstacles on experimental auricular flutter. *Amer. Heart J.* 33:677.
120. RYAN, G. F., EASLY, R. M., ZANOFF, L. J., and GOLDSTEIN, S. (1968). Paradoxical use of a demand pacemaker in treatment of superventricular tachycardia due to the W.P.W. syndrome. Observation on termination of reciprocal rhythm. *Circulation* 38:1037.
121. RYTAND, D. A. (1966). The circusmovement (entrapped circuit wave) hypothesis and atrial flutter. *Ann. intern. Med.* 65:125.
122. SANDLER, I. A., and MARRIOTT, H. J. L. (1965). The differential morphology of anomalous ventricular complexes of RBBB type in lead V_1. Ventricular ectopy versus aberration. *Circulation* 31:551.

123. SCHEPPOKAT, K. D., GIEBEL, O., HARMS, H., KALMAR, P., and RODEWALD, G. (1966). Prolongierte Anwendung gepaarten und gekoppelten Herzstimulation beim Menschen. *Verh. Dtsch. Ges. Kreislaufforschg.* 32:188.

124. SCHERF, D., and SHOOKHOFF, C. (1926). Experimentelle Untersuchungen über die .Umkehr-Extrasystole'. *Wien. Arch. inn. Med.* 12:501.

125. SCHERF, D., ROMANO, F., and TERRANOVA, R. (1948). Experimental studies on auricular flutter and auricular fibrillation. *Amer. Heart J.* 36:241.

126. SCHERF, D., COHEN, J., PARANGI, A., and YILDIZ, M. (1963). Paroxysmal tachycardia precipitated by atrial or ventricular extrasystoles. *Amer. J. Cardiol.* 11:757.

127. SCHERF, D., and COHEN, J. (1964). *The atrioventricular node and selected arrhythmias.* New York, Grune and Stratton.

128. SCHERF, D. (1966). The mechanism of flutter and fibrillation. *Amer. Heart J.* 71:273.

129. SCHERLAG, B. J., LAU, S. H., HELFANT, R. H., BERKOWITZ, W. D., STEIN, E., and DAMATO, A. N. (1969). Catheter technique for recording His bundle activity in man. *Circulation* 39:13.

130. SCHOONMAKER, F. W., OBSTEEN, R. T., and GREENFIELD, J. C. JR. (1966). Thioridazine (Mellaril) induced ventricular tachycardia controlled with an artificial pacemaker. *Ann. int. Med.* 65:1026.

131. SCHUILENBURG, R. M., DURRER, D. (1968). Atrio echo beats in the human heart elicited by induced atrial premature beats. *Circulation* 37:680.

132. SCHUILENBURG, R. M., and DURRER, D. (1969). Ventricular echo beats in the human heart elicited by induced ventricular premature beats. *Circulation* 40:337.

133. SHERF, L., and JAMES, T. N. (1969). A new electrocardiographic concept: Synchronized sinoventricular conduction. *Dis. Chest* 55:127.

134. SINGER, D., and TEN EICK, R. E. (1969). Pharmacology of cardiac arrhythmias. *Progr. cardiovasc. Dis.* 12:488.

135. SLAMA, R., WAYENBERGER, M., MOTTE, G. and BOUVRAIN, S. (1966). La maladie rythmique auriculaire étude clinique, electrique et evolutive de 43 observations. *Arch. Mal. Coeur.* 62:297.

136. SOMLYO, A. P., and GRAYZEL, J. (1963). Left atrial arrhythmias. *Amer. Heart J.* 65:68.

137. SOWTON, E., LEATHAM, A., and GARSON, P. (1964). The suppression of arrhythmias by artificial pacing. *Lancet* 2:1098.

138. SOWTON, E., BALCON, R., PRESTON, T., LEAVER, D., and YACOUB, M. (1969). Long-term control of intractable supraventricular tachycardia by ventricular pacing. *Brit. Heart J.* 31:700.

139. STARMER, C. F., WHALEN, R. E., and MC. INTOSH. (1964). Hazards of electrical shock in cardiology. *Amer. J. Cardiol.* 14:537.

140. STEINBERG, M. F., GRISHMAN, A., KROOP, J. G., and JAFFE, H. L. (1950). A study of circusmovement in human atrial flutter by means of intracardiac, escophageal and vector cardiography. *First World Congr. Cardiol. Paris.*

141. VERMEULEN, A., and WELLENS, H. J. J. Paroxysmal ventricular tachycardia showing fusion with reciprocal ventricular beats. *Brit. Heart J.* (to be published).

142. VIERSMA, J. W. (1969). *Hartfrequentie en impulsgeleiding in het atrium.* Amsterdam, thesis.

143. WATANABE, Y., and DREIFUS, L. S. (1968). Newer concepts in the genesis of cardiac arrhythmias. *Amer. Heart J.* 70:114.

144. WELLENS, H. J. J., and DURRER, D. (1968). Supraventricular tachycardia with left aberrant conduction due to retrograde invasion into the left bundle branch. *Circulation* 38:474.

REFERENCES

145. WELLENS, H. J. J., and FREUD, G. E. Unpublished observations.
146. WELLENS, H. J. J. (1969). Unusual occurrence of nonaberrant conduction in patients with atrial fibrillation and aberrant conduction. *Amer. Heart J.* 77:158.
147. WELLENS, H. J. J., JANSE, M. J., VAN DAM, R. TH., and DURRER, D. Epicardial excitation of the atria in a patient with atrial flutter. *Brit. Heart J.* (to be published).
148. WENGER, R., and HOFMANN-CREDNER, D. (1952). Observations on the atria of the human heart by direct and semidirect electrocardiography. *Circulation* 5:870.
149. WENKEBACH, K. F., and WINTERBERG, H. (1927). *Die unregelmässige Herztätigkeit.* Leipzig, Wilhelm Engelmann. P. 279.
150. WIENER, L., DWYER, E. M. (1968). Electrical induction of atrial fibrillation. An approach to intractable atrial tachycardias. *Amer. J. Cardiol.* 21:731.
151. WILSON, W. S., JUDGE, R. D., and SIEGEL, J. H. (1964). A simple diagnostic sign in ventricular tachycardia. *New England J. Med.* 270:446.
152. WOLFERTH, C. C., and WOOD, F. C. (1933). The mechanism of production of short P-R intervals and prolonged QRS complexes in patients with presumably undamaged hearts: Hypothesis of an accessory pathway of auriculo-ventricular conduction (bundle of Kent). *Amer. Heart J.* 8:297.
153. WOLFF, L., PARKINSON, J., and WHITE, P. D. (1930). Bundle branch block with short PR interval in healthy young people prone to paroxysmal tachycardia. *Amer. Heart J.* 5:685.
154. WOLFF, L., and WHITE, P. D. (1948). Syndrome of short PR interval with abnormal QRS complexes and paroxysmal tachycardia. *Arch. intern. Med.* 82:446.
155. WOODSON, R. D., FRIESEN, W. G., AMES, A. W., HERR, R. H., and STARR, A. (1967). Use of atrial pacing in cardiac surgical patients. *Circulation* 36 (suppl. II):275.
156. ZEFT, H. J., COBB, F. R., WAXMAN, M. B., HUNT, N. C., and MORRIS, J. J. (1969). Right atrial stimulation in the treatment of atrial flutter. *Ann. intern. Med.* 70:447.
157. ZEFT, H. J., and MC. GOWAN, R. L. (1969). Termination of paroxysmal junctional tachycardia by right ventricular stimulation. *Circulation* 40:919.
158. ZIPES, D. A., FESTOFF, B., SCHAAL, S. F., COX, L., SEALY, W. C., and WALLACE, A. G. (1968). Treatment of ventricular arrhythmia by permanent atrial pacemaker and cardiac sympathectomy. *Ann. intern. Med.* 68:591.

INDEX OF SUBJECTS